✚ HEALTH HABITS

DIABETES

+ HEALTH HABITS

DIABETES

A PATIENT'S GUIDE TO CHANGING BEHAVIORS & MINDSET FOR DISEASE MANAGEMENT

JUSTIN KOMPF, PHD

hatherleigh

HEALTH HABITS FOR DIABETES

Text Copyright © 2022 Justin Kompf

Library of Congress Cataloging-in-Publication Data is available.
ISBN: 978-1-57826-919-8

Printed in the United States
10 9 8 7 6 5 4 3 2 1

CONTENTS

PREFACE

FOR AS LONG AS I HAVE BEEN ALIVE, MY FAMILY
would spend weekends in Vermont. I didn't love it when I was
young. There wasn't much to do. There was no cable and when
we eventually had cell phones, there was no service. The radio didn't
have good music either! And the bugs, don't get me started with
the bugs. My great grandmother, Dorothy Yates, lived there until
around 2000 when she moved into assisted living. I have memories
of her serving us lamb dinners, saying "boo" to me, and particularly,
of her opening the bathroom door when I was mid bath telling me
I was going to use up all the well water. This is a long-standing joke
between my mother and me.

She passed away in 2010, and her last years were characterized
by dementia. The house passed down to my great aunt. We would
still visit two or three times per year. In 2017 I moved to Boston,
which was closer to Vermont than Upstate New York. I began to
visit more and grew to appreciate the house as an escape from the
city. Great grandma Yates is buried close to the house. Next to her
is her daughter, my grandmother who died in 1998. I was eight
years old when it happened. The memories of Grandma Yates are

even more fleeting. My grandmother died 22 years ago and as I have grown to love the house something that feels hard to explain has happened. I didn't know my grandmother well, I was only 8 when she died, but I love her. My mom while reading this is inevitably crying (sorry, mom).

Grandma Yates was a teacher, and as my mom tells me, she would write her own stories. I feel regret for not knowing her. She smoked cigarettes and she drank and in 1998 she died from cancer. There are things I remember, or at least I think I remember. Talks of headaches at her 59th birthday party. Not long after, the cancer diagnosis, my mom crying in the park. I ask if she will be able to take me fishing before she gets too sick, we never got to. My family cleaning out her house. The attic was filled with *National Geographic* magazines. I found a cool silver yo-yo that belonged to my great grandfather. I remember her funeral. Great grandma Yates still has her mental faculties. She says no one should have to bury their child. Or at least I think this is a part of my memory. Years later my great aunt, her sister, expresses how much she misses her during a visit to San Francisco. She died when she was 60, without a doubt with many things left that she would have liked to do. She would be 82 now and could very much be alive considering her mother died when she was 95.

I wish she was, and I know people, 22 years later still miss her. When I was eight years old it was a coinflip (an unrealistic one) as to whether I was going to be a paleontologist or an NBA player when I grew up. Most kids don't grow up dreaming to study health behavior change. But that's what happened with me. My grandmother's health decisions led to disease and premature mortality. But that was not an inevitable conclusion. I would love to see everyone obtain the tools they need to take control of their own health. I'm motivated to make sure that anyone who desires to, can avoid a lifestyle related disease. Considering the stacks of research that I have consumed on health behavior change I am the first to say that increasing risk perception is not a great tactic for producing change. If it was, I could just tell you all the behaviors that are good for you and you would feel compelled to go out and do them. If only I could tell you everything that was not healthy, and you'd instantly cut it out, but that is not how this works.

Here is what I can tell you. Someone loves you; I value you, and I want you to have a healthy happy life. I hope that the steps in this book help you clarify your health aspirations, enable you to create a behavior change menu, and provided you with a sufficient option of behavior change strategies that you can use. I wrote this book with love, I wrote it with research, humor, some superhero references, and mentions of my dog Scout (he is perfect). I wrote it as authentically as I can, and I hope you can relate to my voice, and that it gives you the direction you need.

DIABETES AND YOU

Diabetes is a widespread epidemic. According to the Centers for Disease Control 1 in 10 Americans have diabetes.[1] Many of these cases are type 2. Insulin is a hormone that lets blood sugar into your cells. If you have type 2 diabetes you don't respond normally to effects of insulin. Your body also struggles to produce insulin. When this happens, your blood sugar levels rise which can cause health problems such as heart attacks, strokes, blindness, kidney failure, and blood vessel disease.

Treatment and Recommendations

The goal of treating type 2 diabetes or preventing diabetes if you are prediabetic, is to maintain optimal blood glucose, lipid, and blood pressure levels.[2] This can be done with a proper diet, exercise, weight loss, self-care, and medication.[2,3]

Physical activity is critical for managing diabetes. Regular movement improves glucose tolerance and insulin sensitivity. When your muscles contract, they increase the uptake of blood sugar, thus helping to maintain an optimal blood glucose level. This type of blood glucose uptake is not regulated by insulin which is one of the reasons why exercise and physical activity is so important if you have type 2 diabetes. Even one week of aerobic physical activity can improve insulin sensitivity for a person with type 2 diabetes. Resistance exercise also improves insulin activity.[2] Diabetes can be managed with a proper diet. Because diabetes is manageable with specific behaviors, this is not a prescriptive book per say, so much as it is a book that will give you the skills to stick to the route you decide to take. If you decide you want to incorporate more vegetables into your diet, this book will help you think of ways to make sure you stay consistent with it. If you are lacking motivation, this book will help you uncover why change is important to you and help you take manageable first steps.

BEHAVIOR CHANGE MENU

When dealing with diabetes, there will be several behavior change "buckets." categories of behaviors you should be doing consistently. These are our process goals which lead to positive outcomes (i.e., weight loss, reduction in HbA1c levels, improved insulin sensitivity, reduced blood pressure). Process goals may include dietary changes, physical activity, or medication management techniques. For example, more plant-based diets such as the Mediterranean diet have shown success with positive impacts on glycemic control, insulin sensitivity, and HbA1c levels.[4] There are also one-time behaviors you should consider. These changes make up your "behavior change menu" which we will revisit later.

Some outcome goals include weight loss. A moderate weight loss of 5%–10% of initial body weight can significantly improve glycemic control and reduce the risk of cardiovascular disease. Process goals may include consistent glucose monitoring, reducing caloric intake, reading food labels, engaging in aerobic exercise and strength training, eating a more plant-based diet, reducing, or avoiding processed red meats, refined grains, alcohol, and sugar. One-time behaviors may include consulting with a dietician or joining a diabetes education program. Whatever you decide to do is on you. All these routes will contribute to positive health outcomes. The last thing I want to do is paralyze you with information about nutrient breakdown, meal timing, or specialized exercise programs. The important thing is to discover what you want to do and how to act on it.

WHY I WROTE THIS BOOK

In 2014, I was set on conducting my masters research on sticking points in the squat. If you are not sure what that is, don't worry, it is rather irrelevant in the grand schemes of things and not relevant to this book beyond the next few lines.

It was the summer before my second year of my master's program, and as I sat outside the house in Inlet NY that my family rented, that I realized that my research was pointless. Making strong people stronger is great, someone is going to do the research, but it is not going to be me.

I was interested in behavior. Why don't people do the things they should do to prevent disability, morbidity, and mortality? How can I help people change? That was a turning point in my career interest. I switched my thesis to a focus on health behavior change. From there, I wrote about the subject in blogs and research articles. Eventually, I was referred to a personal training organization to contribute to the health coaching book they were working on. The next year, I was asked to write a chapter on coaching health behavior change in their personal training textbook.

While working on my PhD at the University of Massachusetts at Boston, I was given (okay I politely pleaded) the opportunity to teach a health behavior change course. During my first week, I had a wait list of 7 people in a 45-student class. After the first class, a student came up to me. She wanted to join, but said to her friend, "I was going to walk out since I'm at the bottom of the waitlist for this class, but it sounded really good."

I do not say this to be braggadocious, I say this because it had dawned on me that I might have something useful to say. I want to help you understand your behavior and in turn, make some changes that can benefit your life. When I think of changing behavior, I think of the logical steps someone needs to take to get started. The following steps guide you the way I approach coaching.

The processes I cover will focus on the following:

1. **Mindset:** If you do not believe in your ability to achieve or are not ready, you are going to build on a weak foundation.

2. **Aspire:** This defines the direction you want to go in. Who do you want to become?

3. **Design:** If your aspiration tells you where you want to be, the design phase tells us how we plan on getting there.

4. **Execute:** We know where we want to go and who we want to be, we have the way to get there now we just need to put our foot on the gas pedal. In the execute phase, we take action.

INTRODUCTION:
CHANGE BEGINS WITH YOU

I N 2020, US NEWS REPORTED THE 35 BEST DIETS OF 2020.[1] The Mediterranean diet, the DASH diet, the Flexitarian diet, Weight Watchers, the Mayo Clinic diet, the Volumetrics diet, the TLC diet, the Nordic diet, Vegetarian diets, Jenny Craig, the South Beach diet, the Biggest Loser diet, the Zone diet. The list goes on despite the fact that diets for weight loss only work if the dieter adheres to one principle, maintaining a caloric deficit.

There are also more than enough aerobic and strength training programs in existence. These programs also only work if you adhere to one principle, progressive overload. We are constantly being told that one method is the best while being robbed of the fundamental principles that make these things work. It is no surprise that we experience paralysis by analysis. What should we do when there is no clear direction?

Despite our best intentions to be healthy, we struggle. Many of us say we restrain ourselves or try to restrain our eating habits,[2] yet 42% of Americans are obese.[3] We spend 1.8 billion dollars per year on gym memberships that we don't use.[4] Even people who use the gym throw away money with underused memberships.[5] If you consistently adhere to established principles, you will see results. So why, when we have the best intentions, do we still come up short?

REASONS FOR CHANGE

In my first session with Lisa, she spoke about the hikes she loved to do with her husband. I heard pride in her voice when she told me she hiked the most challenging trail in Acadia National Park. She spoke of her love for exercise and the outdoors in general. The emotional, spiritual, social, and even health aspects of her life were good, but we circled back to weight. She noticed hikes were easier when she was lighter. There was a direct connection between what she loved and her weight:

"Lisa, it sounds to me that you don't want any limitations."

"Yes!" she said back to me with excitement.

"Is it fair to say that your health goal is to have no limitations?"

"That's it," she said.

After listening to people, I have found that there are basic needs that being healthy fulfills. People want **balance**, they want **confidence**, and they want **control**. Confidence, balance, and life control are the three good reasons why anyone would seek to change.

Behavioral research and coaching have been longstanding interests of mine. Nearly every day, I am coaching or studying behavior change. They are two sides of the same coin. Research informs practice because it gives us direction in the form of behavioral models.

Models are used to explain the mechanisms of behavior. Under what circumstances would you exercise? Under what conditions would you eat healthy foods? The model is used to answer two questions; **what variables predict behavior** and **how do they predict behavior?** Models are the map to guide action. This book is my map for you.

THE CHANGE EQUATION

In 2003, Margaret Kearney and Joanne O'Sullivan published a paper in the Western Journal of Nursing Research.[6] They provided us with an elegant flow chart of what drives and sustains behavior change.

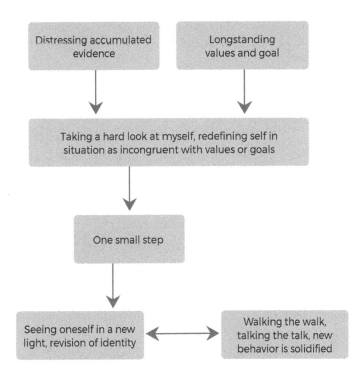

According to their interviews, change was motivated by distressing accumulated evidence. That is, something happened that motivated people to act. For you this may be a new diagnosis or complications that have arisen from a diagnosis. The participants in their study looked at the discrepancy between where they currently were and where they should be. Then they took a small step toward action. If they were successful, they began to see themselves in a new light and their identity was revised.

MOTIVATION SPARKS FUELS THE IDENTITY FLAME

Shirley Webb is an 80-year-old lifter. In a YouTube[7] video, she says: "I'm 80-years-old and I can deadlift 255 pounds. I'm the powerlifting Grandma."

Shirley continues: "I didn't start out exercising until I was 76 years old, and the weights came easy for me. They (a personal trainer) started with my granddaughter first then I was so excited about that, and her trainer looked at me and said I'm starting with you next and right away I was lifting 215 pounds."

"Before I started working out if I got on the floor I could not get up unless I had a chair to pull myself up and I could not climb the stairs unless I used both hands on the handrail to pull myself up. Now I can walk right up the steps and get off the floor with no help at all."

"About three or four times a week my son and I will go my basement to lift weights."

Her son says, "My mom and dad have always supported all sporting activities, so it's turned around where were now supporting her and her adventures."

I like Kearny and O'Sullivan's flowchart, but I have made some of my own revisions to add elements I believed needed to be included. After you look at it, go back to Shirley's story and see if you can notice all the points that are in the flow chart. In the hopes that you will bear with me to explain this spiderweb of behavior, it looks like this:

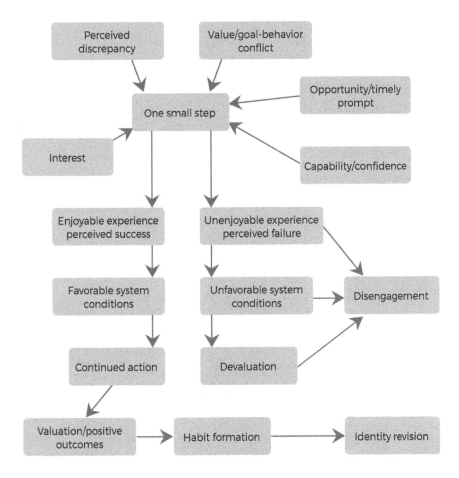

Having a discrepancy between where you are and where you want to be, perceiving a conflict between your current behaviors and your values or goals, as well as genuine interest in a new behavior is the spark that under the right conditions can lead to identity change. If having a discrepancy between where you are and where you want to be is a spark for a single behavior, identity is a self-sustaining inferno for maintenance. If your diabetes diagnosis has motivated you to search for information to make a change, this is a good start. Looking for an answer is step one in the process. You will notice that throughout the chart there are points where people can continue or disengage from their change effort.

This is what this book is about. If you want to improve your health and manage your diagnosis, I want to help you overcome the pitfalls where disengagement can happen. For change to happen you need to be motivated to be different. I don't want you to try to change anything that you do not want to change. I do not prescribe behaviors; I like to let people pick what they want to change.

STAGES OF CHANGE

As you can tell by the arrows in the chart above, change necessitates that you move through stages.

Change means to **"make or become different"** or **"the act or instance of making or becoming different."** I think of change as both an act and an instance. I have been resistance training since I was 16 years old. I can't remember a specific instance where it became a part of my identity but there surely must have been a moment and that moment was not immediately after I started.

Doing a behavior once is fast, but changing habits and identity is slower than most people would like. I, and many people smarter than myself, break change down into stages. To me, these stages look like this:

Stage 1: Non intender

Stage 2: Intending non actor

. . . .

Stage 3: Intending actor

Stage 4: Intending maintainer

. . . .

Stage 5: Identity and habit change

Notice the dotted lines. If you fall above the first set of dotted lines you have not changed your behavior. If you fall in the middle, you have changed your behavior, but you have not changed who you are. Meaning you have not changed your own perception of yourself, and you have not formed habits. You exercise but you don't see yourself as an exerciser. You eat healthy but you don't have a healthy eating habit.

Whatever stage you are in will dictate what you need in a change effort. Non intenders don't need planning and goal setting interventions. They don't even want to change! That's like planning to go to the cinema when you don't even want to see a movie. If you are reading this, odds are you are not a non-intender. Non intenders do not seek out information on how to change.

Many of us fall in stage 2, the intending non actor. You know you should be pursuing healthy behaviors, you intend to, but you don't. You may not be motivated enough. You lack interest, do not have a big enough discrepancy or no perception that problematic behavior conflicts with your goals/values.

Stage 3 is the intending actor. This is the person who has just started a healthy behavior. I picture the road they walk to be like the Bridge of Khazad-dûm that Gandalf fell off while fighting the Balrog in *The Fellowship of the Ring*. Not picturing it? Imagine you are on a narrow bridge fighting a giant fire demon with a whip; essentially defending yourself with a walking stick. AND you haven't even become a white wizard yet, you're still gray. Total bummer. The point is, it's easy to fall off. What is helpful in this stage is a solid **system** that addresses barriers that may be a problem. More on that soon.

After repetitive practice, you get across the bridge and become the intending maintainer. Behavior becomes easier with repetition. Maybe you have been lifting for three days a week for 6 months. Maybe you have been walking two miles three times per week or replacing your morning cereal with a vegetable egg white omelet.

Then the magic happens. One day you wake up. You're excited to go to the gym. You're 30 pounds lighter, and you've signed up for your first 5k. You look in the mirror and see a new you. Your repeated behaviors have become integrated into your identity. Let's begin with two important questions; what do we need to change and why should we change?

MOTIVATION, OPPORTUNITY, AND CONFIDENCE

DETERMINANTS OF BEHAVIOR

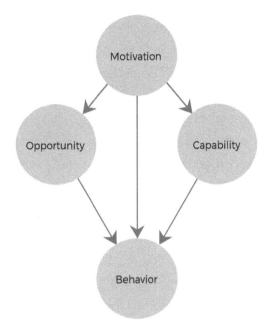

One of the easiest ways to think about behavior is to consider **motivation**, **opportunity**, and **capability**. If you are motivated to do something, have the opportunity to do it, and the skill set to do it, you do the behavior. Dr. Susan Michie, calls this the "Capability Opportunity Motivation-Behavior" (COM-B) system.[8] It is used to characterize and design change interventions.

Capability refers to the psychological and physical capacity to do the behavior. **Opportunity** describes all the factors that are external to yourself which prompt or make behavior easier. **Motivation**

describes all the brain processes that influence behavior. Capability has two subcomponents, the physical and psychological. Physical describes actual physical capabilities whereas the psychological deals with confidence or knowledge to perform a specific behavior. Opportunity has a physical component which relates to availability and resources. It also has a prompt component that is modifiable. Motivation has two components as well. A reflective component and an automatic component. Reflective deals with goal setting, decision making, and planning. The automatic component involves habit, identity, impulses, and emotions.

Miss any of these components and the behavior does not happen. Imagine if you wanted to go for a bike ride, knew how to ride a bike, but didn't have a bike. You are going nowhere. For any behavior to occur, the capability and opportunity to do the behavior must exist and the motivation to do the behavior must be greater than the motivation to do anything else.

If we understand what determinants predict behavior, we can then ask, *how can we enhance motivation, opportunity, or confidence?* We examine the effects of changing these variables. If we change motivation, opportunity, or capabilities, did behavior also change?

There are differences between one-time behaviors and consistent action. Both rely on motivation, opportunity/prompt, and capability but consistency relies on *always* having these three things. It might be a great sunny day (the opportunity) and I may be very motivated to walk, but then not motivated to do that again for a couple weeks. A single behavior is a start, but it does not cause lasting change. No one wakes up, intends to run, goes for a run, and then magically has an identity as a runner and an insatiable desire to run half marathons. It does not happen that fast! Change can happen fast but more than likely you will move through **stages of change.** Next, let's talk about why you might want to change?

WHY SHOULD I CHANGE MY BEHAVIOR?

Don't Rely on Distress: Stop the Problem Before it Starts

If you could stop a problem before it started wouldn't that be nice?

This is a common theme in public health. Prevention is better than a cure. In his book *Upstream*,[9] Dan Heath gives an example of an upstream approach related to crime. Imagine that your house was broken into. How could you have prevented that? Maybe you would have installed a security system? Perhaps even further "upstream" there would have been a program to address potential criminal behavior in at risk individuals so that this kind of crime does not happen. In the case of a diabetes diagnosis, you should not have to wait for complications to occur to act. Don't rely on distressing evidence to get started. Don't put the security system in after the break in so to speak. I would love for you to not need a distressing event to motivate change. I would also be remised to not talk about how great a healthy lifestyle is and how damaging an unhealthy one is.

Why Does it Personally Matter to Me?

When I was teaching at the State University of New York at Cortland, I hosted a day long health and fitness conference. In one of our first conferences my friend and colleague Mark Fisher had us close our eyes. Seven years later I am paraphrasing but this was an exercise that stuck with me. With our eyes closed he said picture your favorite teacher from school and imagine them growing old with grace. Picture your best friend, now think of her father being able to walk her down the aisle. This is why we do what we do.

Why should you change? Health threats do not work well to motivate health behavior change but health concerns are something that needs to be shared. *I'd prefer that you think about what you will gain.*

One of my best training experiences was working with Cathy. Cathy has cerebral palsy, and we trained for three years before I moved to Boston. Cathy is a physical activity professor specializing in working with people with developmental disabilities. When I asked her why exercise was important to her, she told me:

I know it sounds like overkill, but the training is critical to my quality of life. It's easier to fit in with physical activity specialist when they see my biceps before my cane. It's credibility. Personally, I am able to live my life the way I want and not have to worry about 'falling apart' from secondary disabilities, which I should have plenty of. It provides a sense of control over my own health and well-being and that in and of itself is life-changing.

There is not a single person out there who turned their life around health-wise that regrets it. I'm also not naïve enough to think that knowledge of benefits and knowledge of consequences is enough for you to drop this book and purchase a health club membership, but we need to start somewhere! If this at least piqued your interest, we'll move on to what causes behavior and how you can change it.

INCREASING THE ODDS OF CONTINUED ACTION: YOUR SYSTEM

Motivation, opportunity, and capability were all in place and you did a one-time behavior. Heck you even liked it! How can we turn that one-time behavior into continued action? The answer is in your system.

You are a human who lives in a system. You act on the system and are acted upon by the system.

The Social-Ecological Model is used to understand health behaviors and to prevent detrimental behaviors. It recognizes sources of influence as being at different levels including, individual, relationship, community, and societal. These are the areas of influence in your life that make up your behavior system. The individual level reflects everything going on within you. The relationship level represents the people around you, the community level represents your environment, and the societal level can represent a number of things including norms and policy.

If I had data on these four things, I could make a well-educated guess on what you would do. I have a modification of the Social-Ecological Model. The reason for this is that *I only want to include things that you can change.* For example, you have very little control over public policy, but you have lots of control over the food you put in your kitchen. I focus on the individual level, the relationship level, and the structural environment.

The combination of the modified Social-Ecological Model and the COM-B framework makes up your system. The system is my spin on what is called "intervention mapping" which is a protocol for creating health-based interventions.

At the individual level, you have your own motivation, prompts you set up, and capabilities.

In regard to other people, the relationship level influences your motivation, capability, and opportunity. Imagine if a friend prompted you to go for a run, or conversely if you wanted to go for a run but your significant other wanted you to watch a movie. These types of things both affect your motivation.

Your environment is comprised of your home, work, neighborhood, and community. Components of your environment that matter include availability, accessibility, and affordability. If the behavior you want to do is not available, accessible, and affordable, you will have no prompt, no ability, and diminished motivation. These three levels as well and how they impact motivation, opportunity, and capability, make up your system.

If you want to change, think about why you have come up short in the past. Let's say you wanted to go for a walk every other day but came up short. Where is the weak point in your system? If you have weak points in your system, you will experience more barriers which will drain your motivation.

Think about these points:

1. Was it a motivation, opportunity, or capability problem?

2. What source of influence made it harder? The stuff going on in your head (you just weren't ready), your social circle, or your environment?

3. Check off where you think you think the problem may be. When you begin to set goals based on what you want to do you will need to ask yourself "what needs to be in place for

me to be successful?" What you need to change will likely fall in one of the categories in the box below. That is, your own influence over your motivation, opportunity, and capability. Your social circles influence on these variables and your environments influence on these variables.

YOUR SYSTEM		
	Motivation	Opportunity	Capability
Individual			
Relationship			
Structural			

If you check any of those boxes, there is a weak point in your system that needs to be addressed. If you were motivated to do something, but your system didn't support that motivation, you would not act, not even once. Good intentions and massive efforts to exert willpower cannot overcome a bad system.

CHANGING YOUR BEHAVIOR

Change is a process, not a prescription. I am going to share the approach I take to coaching so that you can apply it to your own goals. The first part deals with **mindset**. Mindset is something we have to work on consistently.

Ideally, you will identify the disconnect between where you are and where you want to be. What is your "true you?" Who is the person you feel you are on the inside and how do you want to reflect that person out into the world? Once you have an idea of what you **aspire** to be, you are going to need to set goals. You will set three-month goals. You will **design** what you will be doing consistently three months from now? Will you be eating vegetables every day? Will you be walking or swimming three times a week? Practicing mediation once a week?

Then you make weekly goals. What does success look like each week as it relates to your 3-month goal? Maybe your goal is to do resistance training three times per week, but you currently are not doing any. What does success look like this week? Is it going once? Is it getting a gym membership or scheduling a session with a trainer? Last, you will learn the strategies to ensure that you **execute** the behaviors that will get you to your goal.

The upcoming chapters focus on the following:

First, you need to be motivated. Don't think of this as "Eye of the Tiger," Rocky training in Russia to avenge his dead friend type of motivation, you just need to want to change something! The process of behavior change then involves being honest with yourself. *Only change if you truly want to.*

The process involves throwing away excuses. If you are not currently exercising or eating healthy, there are dozens of excuses you can come up with. The story you tell yourself will have an impact on what you do. You **CAN** do something. The second process then is to *remove the word can't.*

Once you have changed your dialogue, it's time to move to the next phase. The third process is important to get you to keep going even after you have achieved your goals. This is your aspiration. You must *focus on becoming.* Who is the kind of person that would make change sustainable? Who do you aspire to be? What do you care about and how do your goals fit with that?

Next, we design the path forward. You need to set goals. What do you want to achieve in the next three months as it relates to your aspirations? The fourth process is to *set the right goals*. This means realistic, process-oriented goals.

You have shifted your mindset, clarified your aspirations, and set goals. The next process is to build the bridge between designing and executing. You need to find out what you are willing to do. The fourth process then is to *design your change menu*. The menu includes what you can do and what you are willing to do. Achieving your goals is going to be equal to your rate of discomfort over time. If you want to lose 60 pounds in one year, you can do that, it is just going to be unpleasant. If you wanted to lose 10 pounds in a year, you might still have struggles but not nearly as many. When deciding what you are willing to do you may need to adjust the time frame of the goal.

Last, you need to learn how to *self-regulate your behaviors*. How do you make sure you stay on track? How do you make sure that short term setbacks do not have long term repercussions? This is where your system comes into play.

It's my hope that if you can understand the roadmap of health behavior change, what can set you back, and how to overcome obstacles, you can take that fleeting state of motivation and build it into an identity that last a lifetime.

CHAPTER 1

ONLY CHANGE WHAT YOU WANT TO

MEDICINE ONLY WORKS WHEN YOU TAKE IT. THE same is true for health behaviors. They only work when you do them. People intend to exercise and don't, people intend to eat healthy and don't. Outside of working at the University, working with people like this this how I make a living. Helping people close the 'intention-behavior gap' is my job. It is often the case that our good intentions are overwhelmed by our predispositions to engage in bad habits. We have competing goals (i.e., would rather watch television than go for a walk), bad habits, unhelpful social influence, low willpower, and we second guess ourselves. Even with the best of intentions we can forget to do what we intended to do, procrastinate, and miss the opportunity to act.

Good intentions only describe 30%–40% of the variance in health-related behaviors.[1] For physical activity, nearly double the amount of people fail to translate good intentions into behavior compared to those that hold no intention to be physically active.[2] This means that the lack of a positive intention does not explain why a large percent of us do not engage in health behaviors.

INTENTION DOES NOT GUARANTEE BEHAVIOR

The person who says they have no intention to change is perhaps the most realistic. Tell your friends that you are not going to go for a walk, and they will believe you, but tell them that your New Year's Resolution is to start exercising more and watch their reaction.

Jean-Denis Garon from the University of Montreal studied health club attendance in Canada.[3] On average, people believed that they would go to the gym just over three times per week. One year later the researchers discovered that for more than half of the participants purchasing a gym membership is a terrible idea! On average, participants went to the gym 1.39 times per week. Purchasing a day pass each time they went (approximately 5–6 times per month) would have saved them over $300.00.

Godin Gaston from Laval University conducted a series of six studies.[4] He found that only 45.5% of people with positive intentions to exercise acted on those intentions. To some, that might not sound so good. An intention to exercise is slightly worse than a coin flight, but to me that sounds rather good. Especially when you look at what else he found. Only 4.5% of people with negative intentions, that is they did not intend to exercise, exercised.

Action is dichotomous (yes or no). We can think of people as falling into four groups.

These groups include:

- **Group 1 (Non intenders/non actors):** They say they don't intend to do something, and they don't do it.

- **Group 2 (Non intenders/actors):** They say they don't want to do it and they do it. This is not common for health behaviors

- **Group 3 (Intenders/non actors):** These are people who say they want to do something but don't do it. This is common for health behaviors.

- **Group 4 (Intenders/actors):** These people intend to do a behavior and they do it.

Intention is a precondition for action. The energy that comes from motivation drives us to do something, so we make an intention.

Do good intentions deserve such a bad reputation? I would argue no. Good intentions are the first step towards change. About half of positive intenders can translate their intention to be physically active into behavior. Without an intention, hardly anyone is physically active, but the intention-behavior relationship is not extraordinarily strong. The relationship breaks down when people have good intentions but do not act.

As humans, we have the unique ability to think about distant potential futures. As I type this, I imagine finishing this book in a year. It's just as plausible that after a week I could write my last sentence and call it a wash (you'd never know though!). We have the tendency to imagine the best possible futures, but why should we expect what we did last year to be any different than what we will do this year? If you are in the same situation now or a worse one, then why would you expect to be in a better situation next year? Why do we have such optimistic views of the future?

A slight burst of motivation can get a person to sign up for a gym membership. After purchasing it they are feeling good. They're going to do it this time. Then someone comes up to them and asks how many times per week they intend to go to the gym.

"Why, at least three times," they say with confidence.

Where is the evidence that a burst of motivation at let's say February 15th (since that is today for me) will have any influence on what they do on July 15th? This is not to be pessimistic, but it is something that must be considered.

MOTIVATION

Directed motivation generates intention formation. **Motivation** is the sum of all the brain processes that create the mental energy to act. It is the drive to act in a particular way. When I explain behavior change in my health behavior change class at the University of Massachusetts Boston, I conduct an experiment with my students. I ask them to put their hand in the air as high as they can.

Hands go up, most of them still bent because it's not cool to put your hand up in the air as high as you can.

"For 10 bonus points on the midterm put your hand higher." I say.

Hands go up higher. Then I up the ante.

"I will give an A to the person who puts their hand the highest in the air."

Without fail, someone stands up on a chair with their hand in the air. Then I break the news to them that I was kidding and that it was solely an imaginary A.

I enhanced the perception of a desired outcome and motivation increased. There are different types of motivation. In this case my students raised their hands higher for a reward. They were **extrinsically motivated.** In this case they wanted an A, but what if I flipped the script. What if I said, anyone who doesn't stand on their desk and raise their hand right now will fail the class. They would be coerced. This would still be extrinsic motivation though. What I am demonstrating is that not all forms of motivation are equal.

Extrinsic motivation can run the gambit. If your doctor is forcing you to cut out sugar because of your diagnosis, then you are experiencing **non-self-determined motivation.** There is an external coercive force, but maybe you are exercising for weight control, a longer life, or improved health. These are more **self-determined** forms of extrinsic motivation. You are doing it because you value the outcome. If you do something just because you like it, you are experiencing **intrinsic motivation.** If I go for a run in the woods because it is one of my favorite things, I am intrinsically motivated.

Motivation, in any of its forms, is a precondition for action. It needs to be there especially at the start of a change effort.[5] If we didn't need motivation to do a behavior, we all would be doing the things we know we should be doing.

We'd be financially secure, fit, and in the best relationships ever. Essentially, we would be robots! The reality is this; we are not exercising most days of the week and we are not eating healthy. What should we do?

WHERE DOES MOTIVATION COME FROM?

What we've established so far; first, we do not always act in accordance with what we know we should do. It would be nice to be compelled to go into behavioral autopilot, but autopilot doesn't happen until you have integrated health behaviors into your identity.

When you are getting started, you need full attention on your behavior. Next, we know incentive can motivate action. If you were promised a massive amount of money, you would probably put systems in place to make sure you met your goal.

Unfortunately, you are not going to get a lot of money, you are not going to get paid at all, and no one can make you do anything. Motivation needs to come from somewhere else, and that somewhere else is inside you.

Motivation Can Only Come from Within

Picture this, you are rowing down a river on a boat, you look behind you and there is another rowboat coming towards you. You swerve off to the side to avoid the boat and continue to row. You think that you are in the clear, but then you feel your boat being hit by the other boat. You are hit so hard you fall overboard. You are not happy. When you see who was rowing the other boat, you're going to let them have it.

You come to the surface of the water and start yelling at the person in the boat. Except wait, there is no one in the boat. It's completely empty. Where did that anger come from? Obviously, it didn't come from another person, and inanimate objects cannot technically cause anything, **it came from you**. It's the same thing with motivation. No one gives you motivation. Motivation comes from within you. Circumstances might influence the extent to which you experience motivation, but in the end, it emerges from you. What I am saying is, don't count on anyone giving you motivation. This being said, you can be taught things that help you unleash and harness your motivation.

WHAT IS YOUR CURRENT MOTIVATIONAL QUALITY?

Motivational quality matters. It may not be as important for starting a change effort, but it is important for maintaining an effort. There are two forms of motivation: controlled and autonomous motivation. Autonomous forms of motivation are self-determined; they come from within us. We are doing something because we want to. We see value in the outcome that the behavior provides, it is fun, we like the challenge, and it is congruent with who we are.

Controlled forms of motivation drive behavior through sources outside of us. When we are forced to exercise because a doctor tells us we need to, when we engage in a work weight loss program for a cash reward, that's controlled motivation. Autonomous forms of motivation are generally more effective in predicting health behavior change.

Autonomous forms of motivation come from within us. We are doing something because we want to. We see value in the outcome the behavior provides, it is fun, we like the challenge, and it is congruent with who we are. Controlled forms of motivation drive behavior through sources outside of us.

Take a hard look at why you want to change. Do you have a *why*? Are you focused on what you are going to lose or what you are going to gain? Are you exercising because someone told you that you should or is it because you want to be around and healthy for your children and grandchildren? Are you eating more vegetables because you don't want to have high cholesterol, or to take control of your health?

In 2008, David Ingledew and David Markland published a study in *Psychology and Health (2008)*. They looked at how exercise motives were related to autonomous and controlled motivation. Three main motives emerged. They included appearance/weight, health/fitness, and social engagement. Appearance and weight related motives for participating in exercise predicted controlled motivation and health and fitness and social engagement predicted autonomous motivation.

Most people approach a health behavior change because they want to lose weight or because they feel like it is something they should do. That's great, it gets you started, but if you are looking for those results to drive maintenance, you are going at it in the wrong way. You will not achieve notable results in a few months. For example, it takes 8 weeks to build any muscle on a resistance training program. For the person who wants to lose 50 pounds, 10 pounds may not be that noticeable and is not going to happen overnight. It might take months before you can reduce your medication or HbA1c levels.

Think about what you are going to gain. Every time you exercise, you are becoming more fit. Every time you swap out fast food for a homemade meal you are becoming healthier. How can you reframe your controlled motives for autonomous ones? How can you transition from a mindset of what you want to lose to what you will gain?

Think about why you want to change because your *why* is going to be the launch pad for the plans you take on to achieve the results you want.

INCENTIVES AND MOTIVATION

Remember how my students stood up on their desks for the opportunity to get an A? The incentive influenced motivation. There are other forms of incentive. Money is a great example.

What if your job was to be fit? Because money is involved, let's look at one impressive celebrity fitness transformation. When Chris Pratt was recruited to play Star-Lord (yes, yes, I do believe I said I would reference superheroes) in *Guardians of the Galaxy*, he dropped sixty pounds in six months.[6]

If Chris can do it, why can't we? What did he have going for him?

1. A big fat check with the high likelihood (and eventually reality) of a sequel.

2. The pressure of being on the big screen.

3. Career reputation, up until then he was probably best known as Andy Dwyer from *Parks and Recreation*.

4. A personal trainer to work with him six days per week.

5. The disposable income to have someone meticulously make his own meals and snacks down to the right caloric and macronutrient content.

There is the internal pressure to do well for his career, the monetary incentive, and then the guess work on food and exercise can just be taken away. Now the track towards becoming fit doesn't look like this:

Step 1: Become a celebrity

Step 2: Get a movie roll that requires you to be fit

Step 3: Hire someone to make your meals and train you

Step 4: Become fit

Step 5: Receive big paycheck

No, our incentive to change must come from something else. We are not going to receive tons of money or fame, and our career probably will not be on the line if we don't lose 30 pounds, control our blood sugar, or reduce our blood pressure. With big incentives, people can do anything.

Our motivation to act is going to come from: a perceived discrepancy between where we are where we want to be, a discrepancy between our behaviors and our values, or from interest in a behavior along with the perception of a positive outcome from doing the behavior.

DISTRESSING EVIDENCE AND PERCEIVED DISCREPANCY

To qualify to be in the National Weight Control Registry, members must have lost 30 pounds and kept it off for at least one year. The website host stories from successful weight loss maintainers. Their stories perfectly demonstrate the distressing situations that caused them to change.

Registry member Emily Kilar writes: "In 2009, I had a revelation; my obesity was taking over my thoughts, my health, and my life."

Pat Holmes writes: "I am 63 years old and have been a yo-yo dieter all of my life. I have tried every type of diet and support group there is. Finally, 3 years ago I had a poor lab test indicating pre-diabetes."

Raul Robles said: "In November 2009 my wife shared with me her fear that my weight was leading me to an early grave. I weighed 344 pounds, was diabetic, dealing with high blood pressure issues, and, in general, unhappy with my life."

Here are a couple more:

Pamela Holmes said: "I spent 30 years weighing over 300 lbs., from the time I was 29 years old, until I was almost 60. Then my doctor told me that my EKG seemed to show I'd already had a heart attack. That was Dec. 14, 2009, and I weighed 328 lbs. On that day I started my new life!"

Anthony Rocchio wrote: "At 36 years old, I weighed 268 lbs. Staring at divorce and myself in the mirror, I knew something had to give."

You have probably heard these stories before too. They are pervasive in my family. I have an Uncle that almost died from obesity. He was in a coma for several weeks when he caught phenomena. This was a wakeup call. He lost weight, exercises regularly, and loves flexing his biceps whenever he sees me. My Aunt's sister Kelly told me how depressed she was when she was obese. Every day she was putting on a mask acting like she was happy. My Aunt Lisa was overweight and smoked. She felt out of shape, and any form of physical activity would wind her. She changed, quit smoking, exercises regularly, created an in-home gym, and has signed up for her first 5k. Each of these stories strengthens my belief that success is achievable for anyone.

VALUE-BEHAVIOR DISCREPANCY

Values are your core beliefs. They describe what you consider important and can guide behavior. Values have been described as preferences and principles.[7] Preferences impact attitudes. Let's say you cared about cleanliness. You would be turned off by a messy gym. Values act as principles describing guidelines for how you believe you should behave. These principles impact motivation.

One of the goals of Acceptance and Commitment Therapy (ACT) is to increase value-driven behavior. Dr. Evan Forman and Dr. Meghan Butryn work out of Drexel College. They conduct interesting research with ACT and health behaviors. Butryn and Forman write[8]:

Acceptance-based strategies, and ACT in particular, are designed to facilitate the identification and internalization of values and lasting commitment to behavior consistent with these values, and thus should act against the waning of commitment generally observed among participants in physical activity interventions.

In a pilot study to promote physical activity, Butryn and Forman emphasized connecting physical activity to values. Participants in the ACT group were asked to think about why doing more physical activity was important to them. It was made clear that short-term, physical activity can be challenging, and that commitment is more likely to happen when the behavior is connected to important life values. Participants in the ACT group significantly increased their levels of physical activity compared to an education only group.

Clarifying values can help guide behavior, but values are abstract concepts and most of the time are not at the forefront of our minds. If we have not clarified our values, we cannot connect them to our behaviors. Without clarity for what we want out of our lives we aren't likely to recognize a discrepancy between how we are acting and how we ought to act. We feel mental discomfort when our values and actions clash. If you see yourself as an honest person and you tell a lie, you will experience discomfort.

In his book *ACT Made Simple*,[9] Russ Harris encourages readers to identify qualities of behavior in work, relationships, personal growth and health, and leisure. You first identify your values by thinking about how you want to behave, how you want to treat yourself and others. Ask yourself, what sort of person do you want to be? In each of these life categories think about whether you are behaving like the person you want to be, whether your behavior is far removed from how you would like to be, or somewhere in between.

Can you identify some disconnect between how you would like to see yourself or how you do see yourself and how you act? Here is another thing you can do is ask yourself; how are any of your problematic behaviors congruent with your value structure? First think about what you want to change. What are you currently doing that is holding you back?

Next identify what values are important to you. Here is a brief list of some values (again from Russ Harris):

- Acceptance: to be accepting of myself, others, and life

- Assertiveness: to stand up for yourself

- Authenticity: to be genuine, real, your true self

- Connection: to engage fully in whatever you are doing

- Contribution: to give, help, or assist

- Creativity: to be creative or innovative

- Fitness: to maintain or improve physical and mental health

- Freedom and independence: to choose how you live

- Gratitude: to be appreciative of yourself and others

- Intimacy: to open, reveal, share yourself

- Love: to act lovingly or affectionately toward yourself and others

- Persistence and commitment: to be resolute despite problems

- Responsibility: to be accountable for your actions

- Sexuality: to explore or express your sexuality

- Supportiveness: to be supportive, helpful and available to others

The most general link I can think of between values and behavior is that even if there is not a direct connection between health and fitness and what you care about there is an indirect one. You can live more fully when you are healthy, you feel good about yourself, you have less worries, you are clearer headed. Ask yourself if a discrepancy exist between how you would like to see yourself and how you are currently acting.

POSITIVE OUTCOME EXPECTATION AND INTEREST

Social, physical, and self-evaluative outcomes of a behavior describe the incentives people wish to obtain.[11] If your goal was to reduce your HbA1c but did not think going on extra walks would help, you would be disincentivized to go on a walk (for the reason of reducing HbA1c). Positive outcome expectations indirectly predicts behavior through intentions.[11]

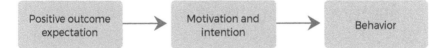

Outcome expectations can be negative or positive. Maybe you think healthy food will taste bad, that it will take too much time out of your life, or that it won't scratch that emotional itch like ice cream does. Some positive outcome expectations you may currently hold include becoming more fit, looking better, having more energy, or losing weight. Outcome expectations must also be considered alongside alternative behaviors. For example, when considering whether to exercise, the option to be sedentary is always on the table.

Having a positive outcome expectation, wanting the result, and having more interest in the behavior than competing behaviors is important. I might believe that jogging will help me lose weight,

I want to lose weight, but hate jogging or would prefer to watch television. Jogging is not the behavior for me.

A final thing to consider is the proximity of the outcome that you want. For example, if the only thing that you are doing to lose weight is exercising more, the outcome you want is far away. Outcomes that you want may also never manifest themselves. For example, if you are exercising to avoid complications from diabetes and are successful, you will never know whether you would have gotten those complications in the first place. The abstractness and distant proximity of this outcome is hardly expected to influence motivation and drive long term change. Rather consider the immediate outcomes, enjoyment, reductions in stress, improvements in energy.

THINGS TO CONSIDER MOVING FORWARD

How do you go about living up to your ideal version of yourself? What makes you want to change? How do you sense that change should happen? How do you identify that there is a discrepancy between where you are and where you want to be?

Goals have a hierarchy. Attainment or performance of one thing is intimately linked to attainment of something else. Guiding life principles are a starting point for initiating behavior change, but they are abstract and content free. Being a healthy person does not describe an action, it describes a quality of certain types of behavior. How do you put your principles or values into action? You do it with scripts, or list of action. Almost like a behavioral checklist. A specific behavior (strength training) involves creating a relationship with yourself, the environment you are in (gym), and the actions you are doing (moving weight).

Let's break it down:

The muscle contractions that you feel during an exercise are in service to the set of curls you are currently doing. You are doing curls because you decided to go to the gym. You went to the gym in service of a goal, of managing your blood sugar. If you have the goal of managing your blood sugar it is in service to the value of being healthy or gaining confidence. Lower-level behaviors are more likely to be carried out if the goal above it has meaning.

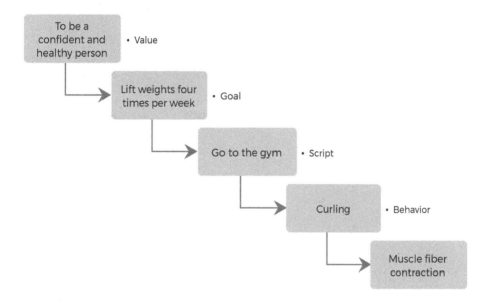

Moving down in level of abstraction and details to ever more concrete behaviors, it is not hard to lose track of the hierarchy of goals that led you to do what you are doing. Abstract values do connect to even the smallest concrete act such as tying your shoes to go for a walk.

What I am saying is; do not lose sight of the forest for the trees. There is a reason why you want to change. The smallest muscle contractions, the chewing of vegetables instead of chips is serving a higher order purpose. Link your behaviors to what motivated you in the first place. Let that be your anchor towards persistence. In the rest of this chapter, I encourage you to consider some things before you clarify your aspirations for your health and fitness journey.

What is Going to Get in the Way?

A client was discussing some health desires he had with me. One of his goals was to lose 10 pounds. He is someone who is healthy so the 10 pounds would be more for aesthetics.

"I go home, and my daughter made this carrot cake." He says "Then she asks me to have some. Am I going to say no to that?"

	Motivation	Opportunity	Capability
Individual	X		
Relationship	X	X	X
Structural			

I've checked off where the weak links in the chain are. In this case the client had competing goals which caused low motivation. The discrepancy between where he currently is and where he wants to be isn't that large. Also, at the interpersonal level, his motivation was reduced by other life goals (to be a good Dad), his opportunity or prompt to eat healthy was not there, and his daughter reduced his psychological capability to eat healthy foods.

Psychologist Thomas Webb suggest that goals fail for three reasons.[12] The first is that people struggle to set appropriate goals. For example, if you do not run at all and set the goal of running three miles every day, you are setting an unrealistic goal. The second is that people do not measure progress. Monitoring progress on an unrealistic goal can be unmotivating. The last reason is that we do not take stock of what resources are missing. I recommend this; ask yourself, are you anticipating how much work it might take to reach your goal? Do you see the time and effort it will take to achieve your goal?

When you say you want to achieve a goal is it anything more than a positive fantasy? Is it detached or attached from past evidence of effort or success?

Researchers Denis de Ridder and John de Wit[13] ask the following questions about goals:

Are these goals authentic or merely a response to persuasive health messages or other social influences that are not well considered and therefore prone to failure?

Which types of goals motivate behavior, and what happens when health goals are in conflict with other goals?

What are the conditions that promote or hinder the successful pursuit of health goals?

Do you really want to achieve a health goal or are you influenced by outside sources? Your doctor? A significant other? Guilt? Shame? Or even fear?

What other goals do you have that conflict with being healthy? If your need for belongingness revolves around drinking with your friends on the weekends a conflict with any health-related goal will exist. Lastly, have you considered how to set up systems that will promote your efforts? Have you thought of what could set you back and removed it?

WOOP

Professor Gabriele Oettingen of New York University has a behavior change technique called WOOP. **WOOP** stands for Wish, Outcome, Obstacle, Plan.[14] W is your wish, it is your aspiration. What do you want to become? Do you want to become more fit? How do you want to become more fit? That is your outcome. Is it as a runner who does 5ks? A weightlifter who can do 20 push-ups? A swimmer who also dabbles in obstacle course races? Maybe you want to change your diet. You want to become a healthy eater, a person who does food prep. What are some of the obstacles in your way to becoming that person? Think about it for a while and write down all your obstacles.

Next, make 4 columns. In column 1, write all your perceived barriers. In the next three columns, write **excuses, barriers that can be overcome with effort, and real barriers**. Based on your perceived barriers, check off what you think it is categorized as. Imagine that I want to become more fit, and I want to become more fit as a weightlifter. I write down all my barriers. They might include knowledge; I do not know how to lift, I do not have a gym membership, I do not know how to write my own programs, I do not have any workout clothes, I feel self-conscious in the gym.

Now let us say the nearest gym is 50 miles away. Not having a gym membership is a real barrier. I cannot be expected to make a 100-mile round trip just to lift weights. Time would be an excuse (for most of us, not for all of us). Time is all a matter of prioritization. If I spend an hour a day looking at social media, I do have the time to lift weights, I just have not made it a priority. A barrier that could be overcome with effort may be a feeling self-consciousness. If there is a gym near me and I have the money to buy a membership, this is another barrier that can be overcome with effort

List of barriers	This is an excuse	This is a barrier that can be overcome with effort	This is a real barrier

EXAMINE OPPORTUNITY COST

In college, I would take my roommate to the grocery store. I had a car, he did not. He would perform mental arithmetic to determine how much chicken he could get for the price of any item. He had the terrible habit of verbalizing his math as well.

For example, I would know that for the cost of a premade sandwich he could get 1.5 pounds of chicken. He was demonstrating what is called opportunity cost; the unrealized flow of utility from the alternatives a choice displaces. That is, if he spends $6.00 on a sandwich that displaces the 1.5 pounds of chicken he could have purchased with that money.

Opportunity-cost means that when we decide between several choices, we give up the benefits of any alternative choice. Picture this, I needed to consume 2000 calories in a day to lose one pound in a week, I could not achieve weight loss and still consume 2500 calories. Weight loss in this case cost me 500 calories. Meaning, I cannot eat that extra slice of pizza and still lose weight. The opportunity to lose weight comes at the cost of not eating pizza.

Whatever behaviors you are engaging in right now, the ones that are stalling your progress have benefits. Make no mistake, they bring positivity into your life. They satisfy a need. If they did not, you would not be doing it. Pizza is awesome. Eating a candy bar tastes good, it gives you immediate benefits. Maybe it relieves stress for a few minutes. Whatever habits or choices are a part of your life form who you are and dictate the circumstances you are now in. If you want to change, you must change what you do. Big goals require big changes. Are you sure you want to cut back on the nightly glass of wine…or two? Are you sure you want to cut back on beers? Fast food?

Make no mistake, there is a cost of being healthy. A person who is healthy does not eat pizza **every night**. A person who is healthy does not drink 5 drinks a night. Moderation is fine, but if you are in a situation where you feel you need to change, odds are that you have not been practicing moderation. Think of the behaviors you do. All of them have some benefit, but which of them also have consequences? These are the ones you must change if you want to change.

Opportunity Cost with a Strength Focus

Recently, I was running in Vermont. If you have been to Vermont, you will know that there seems to be no such thing as downhill. While the distance I was running was short, the elevation makes this run challenging. I got to the top of the mountain and just felt gratitude. I was grateful for my body. I was grateful for a lot of other things that were going on. When I got back to the house, I spent more time working on projects and digitally coaching clients. My day was good, I felt good, and it started with movement.

Psychologist Thomas Rutledge[15] writes the following which is worth quoting verbatim:

People who achieve and maintain weight loss aren't just physically different on the outside or even in the behaviors that one can observe; psychologically, they are even more different on the inside.

These include personal development areas such as improved relationships with food and exercise, new core beliefs, new values about health and fitness, and improved skills with confidence and self-motivation.

Change starts from within, so maybe a better question to leave you with is this. Is there a better way to spend your time? Some behaviors give and some take away. Exercise and healthy food give energy, being sedentary and eating unhealthy food makes us sick and takes energy from us. What do you care about? What do you want to achieve with your life? I'm not trying to blow up the importance of exercise and having a healthy diet, but the reality of the situation is when you have your health in check everything else is better.

CHAPTER 2

REMOVE THE WORD CAN'T

Each day, Dobri Dobrev,[1] who lost most of his hearing in World War II, would walk 12 miles to the Cathedral of Alexander Nevsky in Sofia Bulgaria to collect money for charitable causes. He donated over 40,000 Euros to Bulgarian monasteries and churches and to utility bills for orphanages.

He died in Bulgaria in 2018 at the age of 103. Why am I telling you this? It would seem, at least to me, that Dobri Dobrev had a true understanding of can and cannot. His behavior was connected to such a strong value that he was motivated to do everything that he could even as he surpassed the age of 100. When you say you "can't" do something, keep this context in mind. I believe you have the ability to gain all the resources to do what you want. I also believe we have learned the wrong definition of "can't."

LEARNED HELPLESSNESS

In the late 1960s, Martin Seligman conducted a study[2] that resulted in the term "learned helplessness". For the record, I do not condone this study and it seems that institutional review boards were more lax back then.

In his study, dogs were placed in cages that were either escapable or unescapable. They were given electric shocks. The dogs who could escape the shock got better at escaping, but the dogs who were in an unescapable situation eventually gave up and accepted the shock. Even when their circumstances changed, and they could escape they failed to even try. They took the shock.

Seligman writes the following about learned helplessness:

In summary, experience with uncontrollable trauma typically has three basic effects: (a) animals become passive in the face of trauma, i.e., they are slower to initiate responses to alleviate trauma and may not respond at all; (b) animals are retarded at learning that their responses control trauma, i.e., if the animal makes a response which produces relief, he may have trouble "catching-on" to the response-relief contingency; and (c) animals show more stress when faced with trauma they cannot control than with equivalent controllable trauma. This maladaptive behavior appears in a variety of species including man, and over a range of tasks which require voluntary responding.

Learned helplessness then has main three points:

- Reduced probability of initiating adaptive responses that should bring relief because it has been learned that responses do not influence trauma.

- Challenges in learning that some responses (i.e., escaping) do produce relief.

- Uncontrollable adverse circumstances are more stressful than controllable ones.

In humans, learned helplessness occurs when a person faces negative and uncontrollable situations and stops trying to change their circumstances even when they have the resources to do so.

The person who has tried to lose weight several times, fails, and then stops trying. The person who gives up after an exercise routine does not stick. The person who does not see their blood sugar levels go down after trying to eat more vegetables and goes out to grab fast food. These people have learned helplessness.

LEARNED OPTIMISM

People with learned helplessness think situations are forever. There is nothing they can do. Optimism reflects the extent to which people hold favorable expectations for the future. Individuals with learned optimism think "this is temporary" or "I can do something about this." People with learned optimism bounce back from setbacks. Optimism is linked to good moods, morale, perseverance, problem solving, career success, popularity, good health, and a longer life.[3]

Is the glass half full or half empty for you? When I speak with clients about how the previous week was, they often think about what went wrong. As if 50% success with health behaviors is the same as a 50% on an exam. Imagine if you were not exercising at all and made the goal to exercise two times per week, but only went once. The pessimist is devastated while the optimist sees improvement. The learned optimist also has an internal locus of control. They believe that they take an active role in success.

ABC Model

According to the ABC model,[4] beliefs, not external events cause emotions. Emotions and behaviors are not specifically caused by life events, but rather through the filter with which we interpret these events. This filter is our beliefs. Optimists believe they have the power to change their beliefs. A sequence of events might look like this:

A: Activating event: you eat candy as a response to a stressful situation.

B: Belief: you believe you are the type of person who does not have willpower.

C: Consequences: you solidify your identity as this type of person and do not try any adaptive behaviors.

What optimists do instead is challenge the belief not the activating event. The belief is challenged with a disputation.

"No, I do not have low willpower I just did not set my environment up to make healthy choices. I have actually gained valuable information."

The new consequence is that you do not keep candy in visible and easily accessible places, or maybe you think of a different coping mechanism for stress such as going for a walk or a jog. The irrational belief becomes rational, and a beneficial adaptive response is more likely to occur.

BEST POSSIBLE SELF

In 2009, Madelon L. Peters[5] published a paper in the *Journal of Positive Psychology*. To enhance optimism, the researchers used a technique called the "best possible self." Participants read the following script:

The exercise you will do is to think about your best possible self for one minute and then write down your thoughts. 'Think about your best possible self' means that you imagine yourself in the future, after everything has gone as well as it possibly could. You have worked hard and succeeded at accomplishing all the goals of your life. Think of this as the realization of your dreams, and that you have reached your full potential. Thus, you identify the best possible way that things might turn out in your life. Please, start thinking of your best possible self. I will tell you when it is time to start writing down your thoughts.

Participants were given 15 minutes to write continuously and not worry about spelling, grammar, or sentence structure. They were encouraged to just write. When the 15 minutes was up, they had 5 minutes to imagine the story that they just wrote. Positive emotional affect significantly increased after the best possible self-manipulation as did positive expectations for the future. Negative expectations for the future decreased.

Before we go on, I want you to think about the following:

- What do you attribute failures or shortcomings to? Internal or external factors? If you come up short, is it because of who you are, or the circumstances that you are in? Optimists recognize it is circumstances, not stable characteristics that cause setbacks.

- Do you believe negative events are forever or temporary? Optimists tend to see negative events (i.e., embarrassment at the gym, stress eating) as things that do not last.

- Run yourself through the "best possible self" drill.

YOU CAN

There are over 200 different types of cakes. Each type of cake has its own ingredients but for the most part, they all have flour, butter, eggs, and sugar. Behaviors require ingredients too. For a behavior to occur, an intention needs to exist; I will make intention synonymous with **motivation**. Intentions are essentially directed motivation.

Next, **capability and opportunity** need to be there. In her 2011 paper[6] Susan Michie writes:

> *Capability is defined as the individual's **psychological** and **physical** capacity to engage in the activity concerned. It includes having the necessary knowledge and skills. Motivation is defined as all those brain processes that energize and direct behavior, not just goals and conscious decision-making. It includes habitual processes, emotional responding, as well as analytical decision-making. Opportunity is defined as all the factors that lie outside the individual that **make the behavior possible** or **prompt it.***

The ingredients of behavior change are capability, opportunity, and motivation. Just like how you cannot bake a cake without flour, eggs, butter, and sugar, you cannot change behavior without confidence, opportunity, and motivation.

When a prompt occurs, behavior will occur if ability and motivation are greater than the challenge of the task.

For example, as I sit here writing, my dog is sprawled out on the floor. Scout, the adorable cocker spaniel he is, will inevitably need to go for a walk. He will start whining, pawing at the door, maybe he will do a little pee-pee dance where he curves his body into a C shape and jitters around the room. That cute ticking time bomb, that is my prompt. I do have the capability to walk, so the extent of my behavior will be reflective of my motivation. If I am feeling unmotivated, maybe I will walk him around the block. If I am feeling motivated, I will run the three-mile loop with him around the pond next to my apartment.

Maybe you lack the skills or ingredients to make a Tiramisu cake, but you surely can put butter, egg, flower, and sugar into bowl, stir it then pop it in the oven. You can make a cake; it won't get you on the *Great British Bake Off*, but it is still a cake. And if you keep working at it, you will improve. The point here is that you likely already have the ingredients to do something different. We just need to find out what you are willing to do.

CAN VS. CANNOT AND THE SUBCOMPONENTS OF CAPABILITIES

Only twice in my life have I deadlifted 600 pounds.

I *cannot* do that now. There remains a plethora of other feats that I *cannot* do. I *cannot* run a five-minute mile. I *cannot* bench double my body weight and I *cannot* jump four feet in the air.

However, I certainly *can* deadlift, I *can* run, I *can* bench press, and I *can* jump.

Saying you cannot do a behavior is like saying you cannot ask out a person you like. You *can*, but for any number of reasons, you are just not going to.

In fitness, there are outcome goals and there are process goals. Process goals lead to outcome goals. Deadlifting, the process goal, leads to the 600-pound deadlift, the outcome goal. Reducing calories, the process goal, leads to a lower body fat percentage, the outcome goal. Processes cause outcomes.

Outcome goals are not plausible in the present. You cannot achieve them now because they are in the future, and often far away. Process goals are here and now, and they are plausible. You *can* do them today.

When talking about process goals, *cannot* is a misused word. It sets up a false narrative that allows for stagnation. Yes, with 100% confidence you can go to the gym and lift. Even if it is only one repetition on the easiest machine you can find. Yes, with 100% confidence you can eat vegetables. Once cannot and can are used properly and the right words are used instead ("I don't want to," "I don't feel like it") you can actually choose to move forward to different options or maintain the status quo.

A Clear-Cut Definition of Can and Cannot

Any student who has spent a semester in an introductory psychology class has heard of self-efficacy, a person's confidence in their abilities to execute a task. Confidence in abilities plays a pivotal role in whether a behavior is initiated. For example, even if I wanted to Salsa dance tonight, I could not because I do not have the skills. I could dance or move my body in a way that someone may be able to make an educated guess that I am dancing, but it is not Salsa.

In a 2016 paper,[7] Ryan Rhodes, a researcher out of the University of Victoria, explored how can and cannot are misinterpreted. Participants were asked to rate their confidence level that they could do resistance training two times per week for at least 20 minutes on a graded percent scale where 0% meant cannot do at all and 100% meant definitely can do. After they recorded their answers can and cannot were properly explained.

Cannot was described in a similar way to my 600-pound deadlift or 5-minute mile example. No matter how hard I try, I would have no confidence that I can run a 5-minute mile. Can was explained similarly to the asking a crush out example. The capabilities are there, you just are not going to do it.

Once can and cannot were properly explained, confidence values for resistance training increased. Nothing really changed though, other than the understanding of the word can. They realized they could do it; that is, they have the capabilities. Prior to the explanation, capabilities were considered the same as motivation. Stated otherwise, they had the capability; they just were not motivated enough.

If you have done resistance training or exercised within the last year, you certainly *can* do it. If you have had a single bite of broccoli, you *can* eat vegetables. While the skill set may not be there to do a back squat or make a ratatouille casserole you certainly can do a leg press and eat baby carrots. It might be hard but entirely doable.

Moving on, it is important to properly use the words "can" and "cannot".

HOW CAN I CHANGE MY BEHAVIOR?

Let Behavior Rise to the Level of Motivation and Capability

The first time I lifted weights was with my Dad on some machines in a Golds Gym. I was not lifting astronomical numbers. I was not even skilled. My behavior rose to the level of my motivation and capabilities. I highly encourage people to stop thinking about what they cannot do and think about what they can do. Let's take the strength training example and break it down from something very challenging to something so easy anyone can do it even with the lowest level of motivation.

1. Do resistance training four times per week for one hour

2. Do resistance training two times per week for one hour

3. Do resistance training two times per week for 30 minutes

4. Do resistance training one time per week for 30 minutes

5. Do 20 body weight squats at home during a commercial break on television

6. Do 10 body weight squats at home during a commercial break on television

7. Do 1 body weight squat (go ahead, put the book down and do it!)

With repetitive performance, behavior gets easier. You will not stay at the lowest level of a challenge for long. If you do not feel the desire to progress maybe you were not picking a behavior that was interesting. Changing behavior can be uncomfortable, so you need to pick a behavior that is proportional to your accepted level of discomfort.

Soon, I am going to ask you what your health and fitness aspiration is. However, before that, we need to get in the right mindset. A big part of getting into the mindset is to address the story you tell yourself about your capabilities. I would like for you to have a story about hope and belief, not doubt.

MINDSET

Stop Dwelling on the Negative

"Tell me about your best experience this week."

This is one of the first questions I ask in each of my coaching sessions. I still find it interesting that in the beginning clients have the tendency to do one of two things:

1. Briefly talk about the positive (maybe for 10 seconds) and then launch into the negatives

2. Just launch right into the negatives

In a recent talk with a client, I asked him what went well this week. He could not think of anything. Then his girlfriend chimed in:

"What are you talking about?" she said.

She reminded him that work went well, he got to spend time with his son, and that they were getting a cat! There was a lot that was going well.

Ever find yourself upset? It is tough to focus on anything else, isn't it? You get drawn into your own negativity. What about when you're feeling positive emotions? The world feels like a different place, doesn't it? You feel good, you are hopeful for what comes next.

Rather than dwell on the negative or what you might be lacking, focus on the positive. What did you do well? Positive actions come from positive energy or emotion. Acknowledging what went well can help you build resilience. The way I see it, you have two options when you want to change. You could focus on weaknesses, identify them, analyze them, try to fix them or you could focus on the strengths you already have. Identify how to use them and enhance them.

How can you think of a positive future when you are dwelling on the negative? If you can't think of a positive future, how are you going to be motivated to take action?

Practice Gratitude

Imagine you have a big job at work. You are in charge of securing a million-dollar contract with a company. You make the pitch to them, and they say they will get back to you. For the next few weeks, that is all you can think about. Your ability to focus on everything else is diminished. You are not mindful, and you are not in the moment. You are focusing on something that is no longer in your control. Even when the company says they want to work with you, you still cannot relax until the signature is on paper. How can you bring yourself back to the present moment? One technique I use is the gratitude journal. This kills two birds with one stone. It brings our focus towards the present and is an incredible tool for bringing the positive into the present. Once the positive has come to the present and our awareness is broadened, we can come up with creative ways to address problems.

Here is what I recommend you do. Take 15 minutes for yourself. Ask yourself, what went well today and why? What went well and why addresses strengths you have and positive outcomes that come from using those strengths. Go ahead, put reading on pause and think about this question. What went well recently and why did that happen? This will help to broaden your perspective and get ready to address what you can do.

If I Could Wave a Wand

If I could wave a wand and help a person feel more resilient in their change efforts, I would. I would get them to understand that there is no such thing as failure, only ineffective solutions. Another favorite question of mine is "what did you learn this week?" Finding what did not work can be extremely valuable too. It is naïve to imagine that your first attempt at change will be wildly successful. You are going to have setbacks, but with continued effort it does get easier. You must be resilient in the face of challenge.

Get a Win

When I was on spring break in middle school, my father took me to Gold's gym. I do not remember the individual details of that lifting session, but I do remember catching a glimpse of my pumped up 14-year-old arms in the car window.

I thought, wow, this is great, I should do this again.

So, I did; after school I would lift on the assisted bench press machine in my basement. Eventually achieving the ability to put 45 pounds on each side.

In high school, I would throw together random assortments of exercises in the weight room. Lifting became the tool I used to improve my basketball game, to enhance my confidence, to deal with stress, break ups and to socialize with my friends.

This all began with a look in the car window. I had a win, I had help (*thanks, Dad*), and I had something to be immediately proud of. It was motivating.

Incentives and discrepancies can cause motivation towards action. **Wins enhance motivation whereas losses diminish motivation.** Losses crush what could have been the start of a positive identity shift. This all being said, no matter how many times you have perceived that you have come up short in your health behavior change efforts there is always a win out there.

ASSESS WHERE YOU ARE AND PICK YOUR WIN BEHAVIOR

Below is an example of an assessment of where you currently are in terms of vegetable consumption and in terms of exercise. Find where you are and then if you are comfortable, take the next small step forward. Whatever you pick, be confident that you can do it. Then when you do it be sure to celebrate. Be proud of your change, and only move forward when you feel confident that you can.

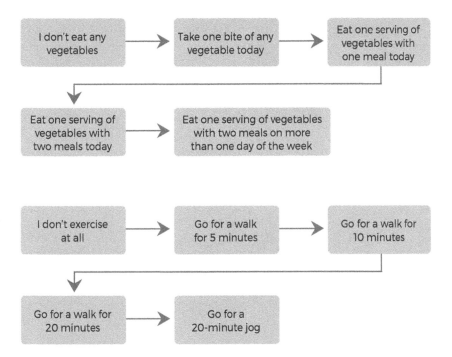

Whatever you pick, be sure to make sure you do it. You want a win! Later, I will argue that there is no such thing as a loss, losses are perception, perception is subjective. However, changing behavior begins with throwing away the word cannot.

CHAPTER 3

FOCUS ON BECOMING HEALTHY

I n the early 2000s, i wrote an "unofficial" sequel to Michael Crichton's book *Jurassic Park.* The novel was written in a black and white composition notebook. Obviously, no one asked me to write this book, Michael Crichton did not contact my agent…because I didn't have one. I do not remember much about the story, but I liked writing it. I kept going back to my notebook whenever I had inspiration for the story line. I enjoyed writing about what I liked. I was 12 and liked dinosaurs, so it makes sense that I would write a dinosaur book. At the time I did not recognize that I was beginning to build an identity as a writer.

I might be decent at writing now and have had the good fortune to be published in academic journals and earn some money. This was not always the case. The first time I ever tried to write for a reputable source was right after college. I mailed in two articles to

Men's Health. They did not get in, and I still have them sitting in my desk drawer.

There were a few things in place that did not let non-acceptance get me down. The first is that I was intrinsically motivated to write. It is not like I had my sights set on a goal of writing a best seller. I just wanted to write. Even now, one thing that gets me into a flow state is to sit down, put on classical music, plug my headphones in and write.

The next is that I was confident in my ability to improve which made rejection fine. I had some blogs accepted on websites, so I had a start. The last reason is that I had a part of my identity wrapped around writing. If you asked me what I do now, it's teaching, coaching, and writing. I am a writer, and I write because that is what writers do. Similarly, I am a person who is healthy, I exercise because that is what healthy people do.

Having confidence in your ability is vitally important. You should focus on what is interesting to you so that you are intrinsically motivated. I also believe it would be a misstep to not focus on becoming, linking your current new behaviors to the best version of yourself.

WHAT DOES AN 80-YEAR-OLD RUNNER HAVE IN COMMON WITH ARNOLD SCHWARZENEGGER?

Before I moved to Boston I lived and worked in Cortland New York. Cortland is a college town. You see the same faces in the same places, and each week I would see this little old lady jogging down the road. "You get it Gladys!" I say to myself. I did not know her name, but

Gladys seemed like a perfectly reasonable one for a woman in her mid-70's.

Two years later, I am back in Utica, New York to run a 15k. Who do I see running along the course? Gladys. Not only is she still running but running 15k's! Why does she do it? Why do so many people try to pick up exercise only to stop?

Gladys ran because she is a runner and runners run. Running has been integrated into her identity. It was clearly a part of who she was and that is why she is doing it.

In 2019, CNBC[1] ran a story on Arnold Schwarzenegger's wellness routine. According to the article Arnold started lifting when he was 15 years old. At 72 he still worked outs every day at 7 a.m. at Golds Gym. Gladys and Arnold have something in common. They both have their habits and routines wrapped around something they care about, something that has been integrated into their identity. If you look at people who have been exercising consistently you can see this to be true.

HOW DO YOU DESCRIBE YOURSELF?

What are the labels you put on yourself? You might start out with "I am the kind of person that...":

- I am the kind of person that exercises

- I am the kind of person that watches what they eat

- I am the kind of person that is good with money

- I am the kind of person that makes sure his significant other knows they are cared for

- I am the kind of person who helps his friends

• I am the kind of person who is a lifelong learner

• I am the kind of person who enjoys the outdoors

Some of these identity aspects are concrete. As an exerciser, I will exercise. If I see myself as someone who watches what they eat, I will be on the lookout to behave in ways that are congruent with my identity. I will build habits around the way I see myself and feel discomfort with behaviors that are not congruent with my identity. If I see myself as someone who is good with money, I might have a variety of behaviors that essentially give evidence to that identity. Maybe I automate money to my savings account, or have an IRA, or practice frugality.

Identity drives behaviors and behaviors give evidence to identity. Behaviors are the only thing that can give strength and truth to who you are. For example, if you see yourself as an unhealthy eater only your behaviors can give that identity truth. The best part is, because behaviors form identity, behaviors can also change identity.

WHO AM I? SELF-SCHEMA

"I am generous."

"I am athletic."

"I am shy."

"I am an overweight person."

What do all these things have in common? They are general representations and evaluations we have about ourselves based on our own repeated behaviors or thoughts. They are called self-schemas.

Self-schemas are our impressions of how we expect to think, act, or feel in different areas of our lives or in different situations. I, like you, change my behavior depending on the context. I may act one way at the University, another way when training and coaching people, and another way when I am with friends.

We have beliefs which form our perception of who we are. It is how we see ourselves. Do you see yourself as an inactive or unhealthy person? As a person with a disease? If you see yourself that way, do you act the way an unhealthy person would act? How you see yourself will be reflected in the behaviors you do. See yourself as shy, you will act shy. See yourself as argumentative and you will be argumentative. See yourself as a fit person and you will do the things a fit person does.

Once a schema has been established it functions in a specific way. The schema we form determines whether information from specific circumstances is important. Our schemas strengthen with repeated experiences. Schemas answer the question; **what would I do in this situation like this?** This self-schema is used as a basis for future decisions and predictions about the self. We can also have self-schemas about our future selves. What are your aspirations? Who will you be when these aspirations are realized?

CHALLENGE YOUR BELIEFS

I was speaking with a new client, and initially she seemed like she did not want to make any changes. After talking a little longer, it was not that she did not want to change, it was that previous efforts had failed and because of this she did not believe there was a viable option forward. This crushed her motivation levels. She was beating herself up, calling herself lazy. I told her to imagine a scenario where she had a personal chef to make her meals, she had a more controlled schedule, and she had a personal trainer to work with her four days out of the week. I asked if she believed that would work for her. She said of course. While this is only feasible for celebrities, the point was to show her that it was not her that was the problem, it was her context. Her thinking and her environment were set up in such a way that there were loads of friction between her and making healthy decisions.

In the context of health change efforts, what is your first reaction to the truth of this statement: "If I fail then I am a failure."

If you believe that this statement is true you are attributing situational challenges to a stable characteristic. Just like shooting a free throw once does not make you a basketball player, messing something up does not make you a failure. It is how we conceptualize the meaning of our behaviors that matter. Problems occur when this dysfunctional way of thinking begins to make it hard to find information that would contradict negative thinking patterns. We only focus on the negative and ignore the positive. From this, negative or maladaptive identities are born.

Notice when negative emotions come to the surface. Choose not to accept them as truth. Ask yourself, "what could be going through my mind that could be triggering or worsening how I'm feeling right now?" Write down what you think the cause is.

For your negative beliefs ask, what evidence supports or refutes these beliefs? What are the pros and cons of continuing to see things the way I see them? What advice would I give to a best friend who has the same beliefs that I have?

IDENTITY AND HABITS

What determines our identity? Part of it is our habits. Habits form when behaviors are repeated in stable contexts. Once habits are formed, the ease with which a behavior will occur increases. You do not need to consciously deliberate what you will do when a habit is formed.

Automatic motivation to engage in a behavior is based on your identity. Identity leads to repeated actions which then contribute to habit formation. The other path is identity based on habits. Identity may develop based on perception of importance. That is if we do something frequently, we may infer that it is important and may be part of who we are.

So, one route in the identity-behavior-habit[2] relationship may look like this. Let's say I love rock climbing. I get excited about things like *Free Solo* and I say phrases like *"send it"* (which I do not). Then my friends start a weekly climb club, which I readily join. I am motivated to do this because it is part of my identity. After repeated behaviors, climb club has become a habit. **Identity-behavior-habit.** Alternatively, let's say one day I am very stressed. Normally I cope with stress by snacking but gasp, I am out of snacks. For whatever reason, I go for a run and that feels good. Over the course of a few months, I run more and more frequently. Eventually running four to five times per week. It is habitual, I have signed up for a few races and have a wicked collection of shirts from 10k races. **Behavior-habit-identity.**

What Type of Habit Should Form Identity?

Some habits such as putting on a seatbelt or drinking coffee are not built on strong values. Nor is it likely that wearing a seatbelt is a pivotal part of your identity. Behaviors are likely to become a part of who we are if two things are in place. If the **behavior is habitual and if the behavior reflects a goal or a value.**

What do you value in your life? Is it achievement, pleasure, independence, excitement, security, kindness, balance, or challenge? If your behaviors fulfill something you value, you probably feel exhilarated, excited, inspired, joyful, curious, confident, engaged, refreshed, content, and affectionate. If these feelings seem alien to you, then maybe your behaviors are only working for you in the short run.

Habits work like this: cue → craving → behavior → reward. We get in trouble with bad habits when we try to rush the reward or quickly remove discomfort. Let's say you feel impending dread whenever the thought of going to the gym crosses your mind. So instead of doing something that will help you in the long run, you have the craving to get rid of this unpleasant feeling. Instead, you watch Netflix on the couch with some snacks. The feeling goes away, and you are immediately rewarded. Rather than being curious and exploring the truth behind your feelings, you ran away from the discomfort.

Take a minute to think. How did you feel this last week? Were you angry or excited? Were you tense or relaxed? Vulnerable or confident? Tired or refreshed? While unhealthy behaviors may serve an immediate function, they leave us in a state where needs are not met. For example, binge eating may fix an immediate issue (i.e., loneliness or boredom), but often causes more problems in the long run.

Values are abstract concepts. Meaning, they are always not at the forefront of our brain. What do you care about in life? How do your behaviors fit into the grand picture of living up to those values? Do you care about managing your health? How does eating ice cream each night fit into your core value for health?

Unhealthy behaviors may be the short-term solution to an immediate problem, but they do not truly meet your needs. Identifying a discrepancy between what you value and how you behave can help motivate behavior. Similarly, identifying a discrepancy between how you act and how the person you want to become would act can motivate change.

WHAT DO YOU VALUE THE MOST?

What do you care about?

Behavior change is driven by discrepancy. Discrepancy describes the differences between where you are and where you think you should be. If the ideal version of me lifts weights four times per week and over the last month I have not lifted at all, a discrepancy exists.

If I see a discrepancy, I will be motivated to take self-correcting action. This discrepancy can be real or perceived. One of the easiest ways to create a perceived discrepancy is to examine how you see yourself. Most people have some area of their life in which they see themselves in a positive light.

Once we identify the best parts of ourselves, we aim to strengthen those characteristics, **not to solve the current problems we have, but rather to outgrow them.** Here is what I mean.

When I was in college, my roommates and I would finish a bottle of liquor between the three of us before going out. That's right, before going out!

The next year, I had a Strength and Conditioning internship at Syracuse University. It was my dream internship. I got up early every day to be there. To still make money, I pushed my work hours at the gym to late at night and early in the morning on Saturday. That year, I did not have time to do the things I did the year before. Other things became more important than going out. Not only that, going out would interfere with the things I found more important. Drinking lost a large part of its appeal.

We see behaviors change all the time when people make important life decisions. Someone has a child; they want to see themselves in a positive light as a parent. They may have to take a good hard look at what they have been doing. How does smoking cigarettes fit into the big picture of being a good parent? How does being unfit and having high blood sugar work into the picture of being a good parent? If you make the decision to set a goal, who do you want to achieve the goal as? How far are your behaviors detached from what that person would do in challenging situations?

VISION FOR FUTURE YOU

Let's say you want to lose 40 pounds. The general direction you will go may include plans to exercise more, reduce your intake of junk food, and maybe practice more mindfulness in your day. You have identified why you want to do this as well. You value well-being, and you care about independence. Who do you want to achieve this goal of losing 40 pounds as? Who is the person that could do this?

One of my clients, a successful lawyer, used the term boss. She sees herself as a boss. She sees a boss as someone who not only takes control but is in control. There is a strength around that word. What would someone like that do in a situation with food temptation?

What would they do when they feel low on energy and don't want to exercise? Rather than solely focusing on the outcome, which in the case of 40 pounds will likely take a year, focus on becoming. You cannot lose 40 pounds tomorrow, but you certainly can act like a boss in every situation. What are you feeling, what are you thinking, what are you doing? How are you putting your values in action?

Design Your Vision

Moving forward you will want a clear vision of what you want to build. Who you want to be should be the kind of person that outgrows problems. If you feel insecure, you might envision yourself as a confident person. That confident person may just so happen to be exercising daily and eating well. A proper vision generates motivation, gets you excited. Visions describe what you truly want, push the current status quo, and build on your strengths. Think about the goal you have. Maybe you want to lose 10 pounds. Maybe you want to reduce your cholesterol or get off medication. Maybe you want more energy.

Then think about why this goal matters to you. "I want to achieve (goal) because…"

Ask yourself if your reason is a strong one. Will it keep you going when change becomes challenging? Think about the following:

- Describe how you would like your health to look 12 weeks, one year, and five years from now?

• What do you believe is possible?

• How are your values linked to this outcome?

• How does well-being fit into other goals you have?

• What would your life be like if you achieved your vision? How would that feel?

Before moving on take a moment to use the sheet on the next page to clarify your vision.

1. Write down a statement that describes the best version of yourself. Who do you want to be? What does that look like?

2. Why is this important to you? What are your motivators?

3. What are some things you truly value in your life that relate to your vision? How does being healthier relate to your life goals and values?

4. What personal strengths do you have that can help you achieve your vision?

5. What are some challenges that may hurt your confidence? How will you overcome them?

CHAPTER 4

SETTING THE RIGHT GOALS

ONE OF MY CLIENTS FELT HIS ENERGY LEVELS were low. The only thing he was being successful in was work. His balance was off. He knew he should be exercising and recognized that he was not where he wanted to be. He struggled with implementation. My job is to help clients figure out what they really want. In statistics, a mediation model includes a third variable to describe the relationship between an independent variable and a dependent variable.

Stay with me; people want to change their behavior not to lose weight or reduce their risk of complications from illness. Even if they say it, that is not the outcome they seek. That outcome is the mediator. You do not just seek to lose 20 pounds; you seek the outcome or the change that 20 pounds brings you.

Let's say you are already within a healthy weight range but want to lose more body fat and improve strength. This is the mediating variable for the real outcome, to feel confident in your body. Our outcome goals are one level up from intentions. Meaning, when we have a goal, we make intentions on how we will carry out that goal.

If you want to gain muscle (the goal), you need to intend to do resistance training. If you want to reduce your blood sugar levels (the goal), you need to intend to exercise.

Goals direct behavior through four functions[1]:

1. They direct attention and effort toward relevant activities and away from counterproductive activities.

2. They energize action.

3. They influence effort and persistence.

4. They lead people to seek out information that is relevant to the goal.

To be an intender who acts, you need to consider the following. One is something you have already done. Be critical of your goal. Do you really want to achieve this or is it just positive fantasizing? If the goal is something you want to accomplish consider the follow:

• What is your SMART goal?

• Why do you want to accomplish this goal?

• Is it interesting and important?

• What is the plan?

• Are your goals aligned with your environment?

IS YOUR GOAL SMART?

SMART is an acronym for **S**pecific, **M**easurable, **A**chievable, **R**elevant, and **T**imely. Specific goals are the exact outcome you want. They describe the when, where, how, and what. Measurable describes the metrics that you will use. The goal of becoming healthier is too vague. How will you objectively measure that you have become healthier.

Here are some examples:

1. How fast can you walk a mile?

2. How many sit ups can you do in a minute?

3. What is your blood pressure? Blood sugar? Cholesterol?

4. What is your weight or body fat percentage?

5. What is your waist-to-hip ratio?

These are all measurable outcomes. Achievable and realistic describe these capabilities. Goals should be challenging but achievable. Do not set the goal of being able to do 100 push-ups in a row if you cannot do one right now. Last is timely; what is the time frame for accomplishing the goal? It is great to have a five-year plan but let's keep our goals in a shorter time frame. I would say one year out is the longest we need to go for health goals.

Process vs. Outcome Goals

Imagine getting in your car. You are going out of town, a snowboarding trip to Killington Vermont sounds nice so let's go there. You get in the car and type in the address. That is your outcome goal. The GPS gives you the specifics, the mileage, estimated time to get there. Sounds like a SMART goal, right?

You are not moving an inch until you take your car out of park and put your foot on the pedal. Outcome goals are the result, it is what you typed into the GPS. Process goals focus on the behaviors you will do.

Here is a worksheet to break down outcome goals and process goals using the SMART framework. Write out the specific goal under the specific column. Then check the boxes below if they are measurable, attainable/realistic, and time bound.

	Outcome goal	Process goal
Specific		
Measurable		
Achievable/Realistic		
Time-bound		

I encourage you to think about what outcome you want three months from now. Make it SMART. Once you are done with that, evaluate what you are doing three months from now on a consistent basis. This is the process part of your goal. For example, if you wanted to lose 20 pounds, you would probably be exercising four or five days per week, grocery shopping with a list, and eating vegetables with at least two of your three meals. Think of the process like this:

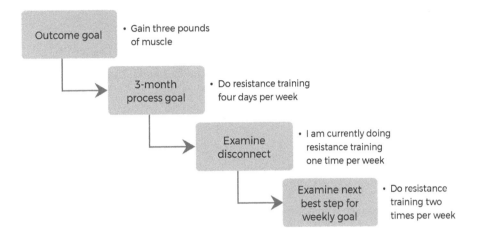

Your outcome goal needs consistent behaviors to work, these are your process goals. Examine the gap between your current behavior and your process goal. How big is the gap? Can you cross it immediately or do you need steppingstones? What are you going to do next week to get closer to your 3-month process goal?

APPLICATION: FOCUS MAPPING

In his book *Tiny Habits*,[2] BJ Fogg describes a technique called focus mapping. This is going to be helpful for your process goals. First, start by writing down your outcome goal. Maybe you want to lose 50 pounds. Next, write down all the behaviors someone who would lose 50 pounds would do. Do not worry if it is something you know you will not necessarily do. Just be creative, write down 20 or more behaviors.

Professor Fogg encourages people to use the following prompt:

If you could wave a magic want and get yourself to do any behavior that would help you meet your goal, what would it be?

Once you have all your behaviors written down, rank each of them in terms of high or low impact. Use the arrow below for a reference. Low impact behaviors go on the bottom. The higher the impact the higher they rise.

Next, we will add a second arrow to make a cross. The second arrow represents confidence that you can do the behavior. If you thought switching over to a vegetarian diet was a high impact behavior it would be at the top of the list, but you have low confidence that you can stick to the behavior it would fall in the upper left corner. If you thought joining a cycling class was something that had a high impact and is something you are confident you can do put it in the upper right column. The upper right column holds the process goals you should be aiming to achieve. They are perceived as high impact and doable.

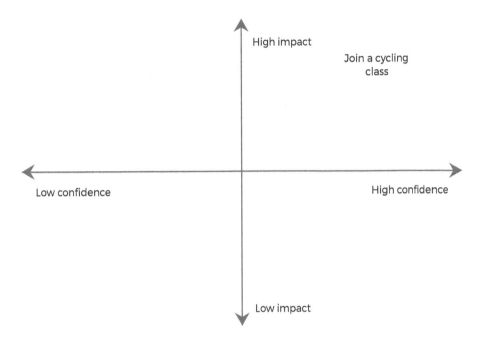

Why Do You Want to Do This?

Let's not forget that your outcome goal is in service of your aspiration. At this point, it is important to make sure the two were linked. If you said you wanted balance in your life but decided your outcome goal was to run a marathon that might not be good idea. Why? Because you would end up running for two to three hours on a regular basis. This might get in the way of other things.

I love this quote from Hall of Fame pitcher Tom Seaver:

Pitching…determines what I eat, when I go to bed, what I do when I'm awake. It determines how I spend my life when I'm not pitching. If it means I have to come to Florida and can't get tanned because I might get a burn that would keep me from throwing for a few days, then I never go shirtless in the sun … If it means I have to remind myself to pet dogs with my left hand, then I do that, too. If it means in the winter, I eat cottage cheese instead of chocolate chip cookies in order to keep my weight down, then I eat cottage cheese.

Behaviors work under a chain of command. At the top of the chain of command are our values. If you value being a great pitcher, then low-level behaviors such as avoiding a tan become meaningful.

Researchers Denise de Ridder and John de Wit[3] write:

In this hierarchical system of self-regulation, a lower level represents the means towards the ends specified at the next higher level, and what results is a "cascade of control", which extends from the most abstract top level at which system concepts (or "be" goals) are represented, such as being a healthy person, down to motor control goals at the lowest level, such as walk to work instead of driving by car.

Values are what we care about. They are the reason WHY you want to put that destination into your GPS. If you want to work on the value of becoming a healthy person, set an outcome goal of achieving a healthy body weight. That outcome goal requires process goals which may include exercising five days of the week. The process goal requires a specific plan on when you will exercise. At the very bottom is the only concrete thing in this chain of command, the behavior.

When you are setting your goal, check in with the top of the chain of command. Do you have a good reason why you want to achieve this goal? Another way to think about your values and behaviors is to identify what is interesting and important to you?

INTEREST AND IMPORTANCE

Let's say I was giving a lecture on how the directionality of time does not exist at the subatomic level (entirely unqualified but I recently read a book on this). Presumably, for most people this does not sound important. It probably is not all that interesting either.

Upon hearing that I am giving this lecture most people would just say "not interested." The people who are not interested are not going to seek out lower-level information. Meaning they are not going to ask me *where* and *when* I am giving this lecture. Location and time are irrelevant.

If the goal or behavior is not interesting and important you will not seek out lower-level information; you will not consider processes or plans. If a goal falls below a certain level of interest and importance, you will join the non-acting intender group. How can you make the process more interesting or enjoyable and how can you enhance the importance of change?

Make it Interesting

Outcome goals are top-level goals. They reside right below values. Outcome goals have multiple avenues for achievement because there are multiple ways to achieve outcome goals. Think about which processes energize and excite you. Think of a behavior that is optimally challenging, where the task demands meet your abilities. Something where you can feel competent and at the same time can gain mastery. Think of an activity you can do that is *intrinsically motivating*, that is an activity where the purpose is the activity itself. If walking for three miles is not interesting what about a three-mile hike? If weight training is not interesting, what about yoga? Find something that is exciting and sufficiently challenging that can fulfil top level goals.

Enhance the Importance

Perceived discrepancy is how importance is judged. Discrepancy describes the difference between where a person currently is and where they want to be. If you have an ideal body weight of 180 pounds and currently weigh 182 pounds there is not a big discrepancy. Low discrepancy means low motivation and low importance.

It is good and important to identify which changes are not important to you so that you may disengage from goals that are not important and focus on ones that are. Consider first focusing on ideals. Are there current behaviors that detract from living up to your ideal self? What is the difference now between actual conditions and ideal conditions?

Next, which of your current needs are not being met? How can changing your behavior change this? If your needs are not being met, you may be feeling some of the emotions in the chart below. Circle which ones apply to you and describe how changing behavior can help you meet your needs.

FEELING CATEGORY	DESCRIPTIVE WORDS	NEEDS NOT BEING MET
Angry	Resentful, mad, livid, irate	Safety, respect, acknowledgment
Annoyed	Aggravated, bitter, cranky, frustrated, impatient, uptight	Respect, autonomy, appreciation, acknowledgement
Upset	Restless, troubled, uncomfortable, uneasy	Understanding
Tense	Anxious, bitter, irritable, overwhelmed, stressed out, nervous	Safety, trust, relaxation
Embarrassed	Ashamed, hesitant, lost, torn	Appreciation, to be seen, autonomy
Longing	Envious, yearning	Belonging, acknowledgment, connection, community
Tired	Beat, burned out, depleted, weary, worn out	Relaxation, balance
Sad	Depressed, disappointed, unhappy	Support, understanding

EFFORT OR CAPABILITY?

Challenging goals cannot be achieved without overcoming barriers. Belief in ability to succeed and having a strong sense of self-efficacy is vital for success. Progress towards a goal can be thwarted by one of two things, lack of capabilities or lack of effort. If capability was the issue the process goal was too challenging. Most people have the capability to engage in health-related behaviors. Certainly, some health-related behaviors are more challenging than others and often require skill. For example, the deadlift is a technical exercise that not everyone has the capability to complete with correct form. However, with a few exceptions, most people have the capability to do resistance training.

People may not have the capability to run a seven-minute mile, but they do have the capability to go on a walk for 10 minutes. Process goals that are challenging but matched for current capabilities should have already been set. If appropriate process goals are set, shortcomings are a result of a lack of effort. This could be for several reasons. Maybe the goal was not interesting and important. If that was the case, review the section on goal hierarchy.

Self-efficacy is important because people with high self-efficacy consider shortcomings to be a result of insufficient efforts. They evaluate and then increase effort and persistence when they come up short. People with low self-efficacy attribute their failures to low ability.

Perceived inability is caused by one of four things: **time, physical effort, mental effort,** or **money.** Inability due to lack of perceived time is a priority issue. You do not have a lack of time to be healthy. If you are eating, you had time to eat something healthier. If you watched an hour of Netflix, you had time to exercise (you can also exercise and watch Netflix). Your goal was just not a priority. Physical and mental effort are interconnected. If the task ahead is too physically daunting, it probably has a mental effect too. Even the thought of five hours of food prep is mentally draining. Let alone the clean up! Exercising seven days a week for an hour seems similarly physically daunting. If you are doing nothing at the current moment, do not imagine you need to take such giant steps forward. Start slow.

Without a doubt, money is a real issue. If you had millions of dollars, you would have a personal trainer and personal chef. You wouldn't even have to rely on motivation. For some, the $50.00 per month for a gym membership may be too much. But then again, I would ask you about priorities. Did you buy new clothes this month? How many times did you go out to eat? If you don't have money to spare, don't worry. Exercise is free. There are hundreds of body weight exercises you can do, and jogging happens to be free as well.

WHAT CAN I DO THAT I AM WILLING TO DO?

As a disclaimer, there *are* real "cannots." You cannot do a back squat unless you have a gym membership or a squat rack. Nor can you go for a run without running shoes. Limitations are real, but only exclude a small percent of us from exercise and improvement.

"What can I do?" is going to be the first question, immediately followed by "what am I willing to do?"

Goals necessitate a willingness to change. An opportunity-cost will always exist in a change effort. What am I willing to give up to get what I want? Drinking 30 beers a week is counterproductive to a weight loss goal. Opportunities have a cost. If you are lifting weights for 30 minutes you cannot simultaneously be watching Netflix on your couch for 30 minutes.

If you are not willing to give on something, be honest with yourself, it is a motivation issue not a capability issue. That is fine if that is the case. If you aspire to be healthier and manage your diabetes, there are a lot of things you can change. If something does not sound appealing just move on to another option. If you are willing to change something, then it is time to design your change menu.

DESIGN YOUR CHANGE MENU

Your change menu is composed of what you can do AND what you are willing to do. If you do not know how to do certain exercises it cannot be on your menu. Your menu would need to say "learn how to do X, Y, Z" instead.

If you do not know how to write your own fitness program, you cannot say "write my own fitness program." It needs to be "hire someone to write my program" or "hire someone to teach me to write a program."

If you can do it, what are you willing to do? How much time are you willing to dedicate to it?

If you can jog, what are you willing to do? How far, how fast, how many days?

If you can lift, what are you willing to do? What exercises, how long, how many days?

For the most part, we are entirely capable of doing the things that would lead us to reach our goals. We *can* cut calories. We *can* push ourselves to lift heavier, to learn new exercises. We *can* persist year in and year out. Match your goals to what you are willing to put on your change menu.

I realize it's just vernacular, but it's words that tell us the story we follow. It is rarely an issue of if you *can* do it. Arguably, most reasonable fitness goals can be chipped away at with time and persistence. It is all a matter of picking what you can do right now and choosing goals that match what you are willing to do.

CHAPTER 5

CREATING YOUR CHANGE MENU

Discomfort is the absence of comfort or ease. It is anything that interferes with comfort. Make no mistake, change can cause discomfort. Not extreme pain, not extreme hardship, but some mild amount of it. Whether it is from a caloric deficit, feeling uncomfortable in the gym, walking an extra ten minutes, or doing one more rep on a machine, you will experience some discomfort.

WHY THE HECK DOES PELOTON WORK?

I was on the phone with one of my clients discussing metrics for consumer satisfaction for my dissertation website. He is a venture capitalist who has investments in fitness technology, so I wanted to get his insight. The goal of my research is to get novices to strength train.

"So, the goal is to get people who don't do resistance training to do resistance training?" he asks. A bit tangentially to the research he goes on "that's a good question, so like why the hell does Peloton work?"

"I am assuming because it's fun, right?" I say.

"You know, when they pitched it to us, I was like, so people will sit in the basement and go on a bike and take classes, and I was like, this will never work. And you know, if you asked me again now, I would still pass on it, but it worked and why did it work?"

This client is a data guy. He has invested in a wearable tech company that measures and tracks recovery. Initially I thought they would be a completely different target audience.

"I would imagine Peloton inspires new people because it is fun, and your tech gets the more hardcore person?" I asked

"You know, it's almost a perfect overlap in customers" he told me.

I found that fascinating. "What do you think they buy first?" I asked?

"Oh, most likely the Peloton."

This was interesting to me. Something that was fun might get people hooked to exercise. Once they find a way that they like to exercise, then they start investing in learning more about their health and fitness.

Motivation leads to a small step, a small step leads to multiple small steps if the **experience is enjoyable, fun, or satisfying.** It needs to elicit positive emotion as a reward. The first step needs to be something that makes you feel good.

However, it cannot just be the reward that is good. It needs to be that the reward is better than any experienced discomfort. Exercise has an affective component, the feeling part, and it doesn't always feel great at first. If exercise felt so good and if eating vegetables gave the same reward response as candy, everyone would be healthy. So, something needs to feel good, despite something else not so good.

DESIGNING YOUR CHANGE MENU

Designing your behavior change menu has some caveats:

1. **Pick something that you find fun and/or interesting.**

2. **Rate of change is a function of the rate of discomfort experienced.** If you wanted to lose 20 pounds in 2 months you certainly could do it. It would be uncomfortable. To lose 10 pounds in 2 months would be less uncomfortable.

3. **The best choice for changing your behavior needs to be a function of your accepted level of discomfort**. If you are not okay with feeling a certain level of emotional or physical discomfort, then tone it down. Find what you can accept.

4. **If you cannot accept some level of discomfort, you are not ready to change. We strive for the path of least resistance but that does not mean it won't be tough for a little while.**

DISCOMFORT AS AN INDICATOR OF CHANGE

Each morning I take the T into work. As I wait for the train, I'm serenaded by a Fred Astaire impersonator, a man in his fifties holding a microphone. He slowly moves side to side as he sings.

I would be less than thrilled to sing karaoke in a bar and would rather eat live bees than sing in a subway station to an audience, mildly captivated for as long takes for their train to arrive. The Fred Astaire impersonator needs to be okay knowing that people are going to think he is a little odd. He is going to have to be okay being out of place. He stands out like a sore thumb, no one else is singing decades old show tunes at 7:00am, and I find myself thinking how uncomfortable this would be for me to do.

There was no way he was exuding confidence the first time he did his act. Walking down the Harvard Square ramp for the first time, I imagine him being at least a little bit nervous. He did not seem nervous today. He looked like he was having a good time. He was not even collecting money. He was doing it for fun.

We all aspire to be something. Maybe subway singing is not your jam but there is something you want to do that you are not doing. Doing something new and becoming proficient typically involves some sort of struggle.

Two Types of Discomfort

There are two different types of discomfort: emotional and physical. Emotional discomfort is that nasty voice in your head telling you that you are looking foolish or telling you that change is not worth it. Emotional discomfort pushes us away from trying new things. It demotivates us. Physical discomfort is what you experience on the last few repetitions of a tough set or the last five minutes of a jog. It is what you feel when you have not had a meal in a while. It directs behavior. It tells us to stop (i.e., stop running) or it tells us to do something (eat food).

Here is an exercise example:

>   **Emotional discomfort**: You feel foolish trying to work an
>   exercise machine.
>
>   **Physical discomfort**: You start a jog, and it does not feel good.

Here is a dietary example:

>   **Emotional discomfort**: You are stressed and want to cope by
>   eating.
>
>   **Physical discomfort**: Your tummy is rumbling.

Is discomfort holding you back from action or is it preventing you from taking further action? What kind of discomfort is holding you back?

EMOTIONAL DISCOMFORT

You need to be okay with putting your head in the butt seat. Yes, you need to be okay with putting your head in the butt seat. Meaning, you need to be okay not being perfect the first time you try changing your behavior.

We try to present ourselves in ways that minimize or omit undesired characteristics. We want to be seen in a positive light. We want to put our best self out there for the world to see. It gets uncomfortable when we do not seem like we know what we are doing. Comedian Kevin Hart made a great joke about this. It went like this:

I don't know how to use the equipment either...I was trying to work my legs the other day—you know the leg machine where you sit there and go like (references leg extension machine). Well, I get there, and it was reclined down, like it was all flat on one level, so I thought it was arms. So, I was like okay, I'm gonna work my arms. My face was burning and everything. So, I'm doing something right. So, I got up and some guy sat down right where my face was. I was like hey man, I was trying to tell him, you are doing it wrong, it's arm. He said no, it's legs...I was so pissed off because I did three sets. He watched me do three sets!

What starts with confusion and frustration (putting your head in the butt seat) does not stay like that if you stick with it. Unless you are training at home, physical activity occurs in social contexts, it seems reasonable that self-presentational strategies would have an impact on exercise participation. It is easy for a fit person to go into the gym because they are reflecting fitness, but what does a novice perceive that they reflect? If it is simply a lack of skill or ability, why would they want to put that on display?

We do not want to be evaluated negatively. Negative physique-related perceptions can prompt protective self-presentational behaviors which deter people from being physically active in the first place. Social anxiety describes an affective consequence experienced when people doubt their ability to make a good impression on others.

Social physique anxiety is this sense of anxiety in relation to your body type in an exercise setting. The gym is a social setting where many people believe they are putting their body, physical prowess, and skills in front of a stage of their peers. Similarly, with weight loss efforts we do not like to feel like we are failing.

Reducing body weight is challenging and slow. This slowness can make us feel like failure. Even greater negativity will be felt when the scale does not move after a few weeks. Lack of results makes us feel like we are just no good. The simplest way to get rid of these negative feelings is to stop. Stress eating, behavioral inhibition, depression can all make us fall off the wagon and relapse to unhealthy habits.

THE TRUTH OF NEGATIVE THOUGHTS

The sun revolves around the earth, 2 plus 2 is four, and my dog, Scout will love you forever if you give him bacon. These are things that are true.

Thoughts on the other hand do not live in the physical realm. They live in the electrical impulses in your brain that give rise to thought. They are only true if actions make them true. If an unpleasant emotional though pops up "I am a failure," "I cannot commit," "I look dumb and out of place," you are the only one who can make it true. What I would do is examine the **workability** of that thought.

Workability means if I accept this thought as true will it help me reach my goals? If the answer is no, reject that thought like a friend request from your crazy ex and move on with your awesome life.

EMOTIONAL DISCOMFORT
AND THE HABIT LOOP

Over the course of two recent coaching calls my clients discussed unwanted behaviors that were caused by urges or feelings. One client said she was normally great at coping with stress. But in some circumstances, she has triggers that take her over the edge. The triggers culminate in anger and stress. Anger and stress resulted in a desire to eat unhealthy food.

Emotions are one of the triggering events for a habitual response. Particularly, an urge that leads to a habitual response.

In this case, this client's habit looked like this:

Trigger: Anger and stress

Urge: To eat unhealthy food

Behavior: Eat unhealthy food

Reward: The food taste good

Emotion related triggers are much harder to change than environmental triggers. For example, if a trigger to eat candy was seeing candy in the pantry, getting rid of the candy would be an easy way to break that habit loop. Emotions are more challenging.

Let's think about it this way. Something happens in your day and your body makes an emotion. Maybe you felt you were criticized, you feel overworked, pressure, taken for granted. Whatever is going on, you feel a negative emotion. This likely means that some need is not being met. Maybe you were criticized and that made you feel embarrassed or filled you with anxiety. Your go to response when that happens is to stop by the fast-food joint on the way home. It is comfort food for you, but is that really helping you meet your needs?

Your emotional trigger is telling you something. In order to break the habit loop, think of alternative behavior responses to emotional discomfort. Responses should ideally get at the heart of what need is not being met. That will provide the reward and help to reinforce a healthier behavioral option.

COPING WITH PHYSICAL DISCOMFORT

Physical discomfort is different than emotional discomfort. While the emotional discomfort of resisting impulses for food or feeling down when the scale does not move lives in your head, hunger is a very physical thing. So is the stress put on your body during a run or heavy squat.

We need to accept physical discomfort and modulate it. Not eating for four days straight would be extremely physically discomforting, you would of course lose weight, but it would not be smart. Similarly putting 315 pounds on a squat would not be wise for a novice. The stimulus is too great.

We need to be okay with some level of discomfort. If you had the ability to do ten repetitions on a certain exercise you would begin to feel discomfort on the second or third rep. The intensity of the discomfort would increase as you continued. You could stop, to the detriment of your goals or you could keep going. You might feel hunger after not eating for a few hours. This does not mean you need to eat every time your tummy rumbles.

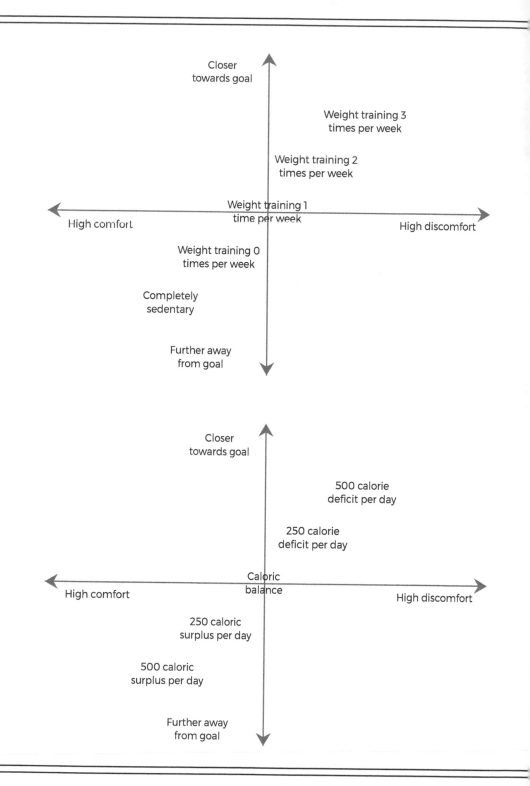

Take a look at the charts on the previous page. Each day your behaviors will put you in one of three categories:

- **Goal achieving:** You are moving closer to your goal. You are experiencing some discomfort.

- **Neutral:** You stay the same.

- **Goal thwarting:** You are moving further away from a goal. You are in a state of constant comfort.

The human body is an incredible thing. It adapts. If you were currently doing resistance training one time per week, going up to four times per week would be extremely uncomfortable! If you went to the gym two times per week, you would experience some initial discomfort, but after a few weeks, that discomfort would no longer exist. Your benchmark for what is uncomfortable will change. This is good! This means that you are changing. You used to find an 12:00 minute mile to be an all-out effort, now you can keep that 10:00 minute/mile pace for three miles. You adapt which is why it is not necessary to rush the discomfort process.

Review the table on the following page. Using it as a tool, figure out where you are now and think of the next few logical steps. Then pick which behavior you are ready to jump to. Remember, the bigger the change the harder it is and the less likely it is to stick, so choose wisely. Conversely, if you went too big at first, make a smaller change. Pick three or four good things you are doing and then identify what a minor, moderate, and major change may look like.

Behaviors	Minor change	Moderate change	Major change

The previous chapter asked you to throw away the word "can't." It encouraged you to understand that there is something you can do. This chapter focuses on what you are willing to do. If you wanted to get to a town 10 miles away, are you willing to sprint there? You would get there fast, but it would be extremely uncomfortable (and physiologically impossible). Or do you want to walk there? Do you want to walk there and maybe take a pit stop? You still have to do the work, but it will be less uncomfortable, and it will take longer.

BASIC PSYCHOLOGICAL NEED SATISFACTION

Much like how we need food, shelter, and water to survive, we have psychological needs that must be met to thrive. If any of your needs are not satisfied you likely will not persist with the healthy behavior you are trying to adopt. Humans three basic psychological needs include relatedness, competency, and autonomy. For this section I will focus on competency and autonomy. Richard Ryan and Edward Deci[1] state the following:

Feelings of effectance nourish people's selves, whereas feelings of ineffectance threaten their feelings of agency and undermine their ability to mobilize and organize action. Thus, to develop a true sense of perceived competence, people's actions must be perceived as self-organized or initiated; in other words, people must feel ownership over the activities at which they succeed.

We need to feel successful, and we need to feel like we want to do the things we are successful at. For example, you might be great at your job but hate going there every day. You do not feel autonomy. Autonomy, when satisfied enhances competency. Autonomy is self-endorsement of a behavior.

The point is to pick things that you want to do. There is no direct route towards health and fitness. For me, lifting weights and the occasional run is my route. For someone else it might be running and rock climbing. For another person it might be dancing, or it could be yoga.

When our needs are met, we may experience intrinsic motivation, internalization, and/or integration. These concepts are going to be important for long term persistence of a behavior. When you experience **intrinsic motivation**, you engage in a behavior because it is satisfying, it is enjoyable, and you want to do it. You do not need external reasons to do it. **Internalization** refers to valuing the activity or the outcome and **integration** describes when a behavior has become a part of who you are. I say all of this because these are our end goals. If we want to persist, we must do the following:

• **Accept some level of discomfort.** The key is to pick the right amount, the amount you can accept.

• **Pick what matters.** This means, your behavior change menu should be comprised of things you feel that you can improve upon (competency) and things you want to do (autonomy).

BEHAVIOR CHANGE MENU OPTIONS

If you are not sure where to start, take a look at this behavior change menu. Treat this just like a menu at a restaurant. Only pick what you want to do. Then pick the appropriate portion.

BEHAVIOR CHANGE MENU			
Exercise and Physical Activity	**Diet and Weight**	**Life and Energy**	**Sleep**
· Take the stairs whenever applicable	· Reduce soda intake	· Spend more time with loved ones	· Go to bed 30 minutes earlier
· Take a 10-minute walk	· Weigh yourself daily	· Consistently take medication	· Avoid caffeine in the afternoon
· Add strength training to your routine	· Include green vegetables to meals	· Cut out toxic relationships	· Keep a consistent sleep schedule
· Add aerobic training to your routine	· Avoid trigger-based eating (stress)	· Don't judge others	· Shut off electronics one hour before bed
· Walk 10,000 steps per day	· Keep a diet journal or track food intake	· Start a gratitude journal	· Cut back on alcohol
· Go hiking once per week	· Meal prep once per week	· Write a gratitude letter	· Cut down on TV time
· Do body weight exercises during commercial breaks	· Replace starchy carbohydrates with vegetables	· Practice meditation	
· Get outside more frequently	· Do not multitask when you eat	· Unplug from social media	
	· Have a fruit smoothie for breakfast	· Treat yourself (i.e., pedicure, massage)	
	· Reduce eating out by one time per week	· Monitor blood sugar	
	· Read food labels		
	· Cut down on processed meats		

YOUR BEHAVIOR CHANGE MENU

Before you move to the next section let's solidify your menu. We are going to write down three to five things that we want to be doing consistently. These things need to match with your goals, be something you feel confident you can do, and be something you want to do. If your behaviors do not match with your goals do not do it. If you do not feel confident you can do the behavior (lower than an 8) reduce the task demand (make it easier). If you picked something you do not want to do (lower than an 8), think of something else.

MY BEHAVIOR CHANGE MENU			
Behavior	Will this behavior have an impact on my goals?	How confident am I that I can do this behavior (1-10)	How willing am I to do this behavior now (1-10)

Before you move to the next section, take your behavior change menu and plug it into the worksheets below. First, write down your health and fitness aspiration. Who do you want to become? Then write down your 3-month goal. Maybe it is to lose 20 pounds, reduce your blood sugar, blood pressure, or waist to hip ratio. In the week 1 goals column write down your process goals from the behavior change menu. At the end of the week revisit it. Rank your perception of success for each behavior and then write down what you learned. In the last chapter, you will learn about techniques to help you stick with whatever plan you make. If you run into barriers, examine them, and then pick the right technique to increase your odds of success the next week. Repeat this for 3-months and assess what your next outcome goal is.

HEALTH AND FITNESS ASPIRATION		
3-Month goal:		
Week 1 Goals	Percent of perceived success	What did I learn?

HEALTH AND FITNESS ASPIRATION		
3-Month goal:		
Week 2 Goals	Percent of perceived success	What did I learn?

HEALTH AND FITNESS ASPIRATION		
3-Month goal:		
Week 3 Goals	Percent of perceived success	What did I learn?

HEALTH AND FITNESS ASPIRATION		
3-Month goal:		
Week 4 Goals	Percent of perceived success	What did I learn?

HEALTH AND FITNESS ASPIRATION		
3-Month goal:		
Week 5 Goals	Percent of perceived success	What did I learn?

HEALTH AND FITNESS ASPIRATION		
3-Month goal:		
Week 6 Goals	Percent of perceived success	What did I learn?

HEALTH AND FITNESS ASPIRATION		
3-Month goal:		
Week 7 Goals	Percent of perceived success	What did I learn?

HEALTH AND FITNESS ASPIRATION		
3-Month goal:		
Week 8 Goals	Percent of perceived success	What did I learn?

HEALTH AND FITNESS ASPIRATION		
3-Month goal:		
Week 9 Goals	Percent of perceived success	What did I learn?

HEALTH AND FITNESS ASPIRATION		
3-Month goal:		
Week 10 Goals	Percent of perceived success	What did I learn?

HEALTH AND FITNESS ASPIRATION		
3-Month goal:		
Week 11 Goals	Percent of perceived success	What did I learn?

HEALTH AND FITNESS ASPIRATION		
3-Month goal:		
Week 12 Goals	Percent of perceived success	What did I learn?

CHAPTER 6

EXECUTING YOUR PLAN

THIS IS WHERE WE PUT IT ALL TOGETHER. YOU have identified behaviors you want to do that are interesting to you. They are based on your values and goals. You are in the right mindset, and you have sufficient motivation to start. The strategies that you are going to learn here will help you follow through on your good intentions. These strategies describe how to hack your system to fix any weak link you may have.

MOTIVATION, CAPABILITY, AND OPPORTUNITY

In her 2011 paper,[1] in Implementation Science, Dr. Susan Michie provided us with definitions of motivation, capability, and opportunity. **Motivation** is defined as all the brain processes that energize and direct behavior. This covers automatic processes as well as choice and intention. It includes habit, emotional responding, and analytical decision making. We can think of motivation in a deliberate intentional way, and we can think of motivation in an automatic more habitual way. In her book, *Good Habits, Bad Habits*,[2] Dr. Wendy Wood considers habits to be "automaticity in lieu of conscious motivation". **Capability** is a person's psychological and physical capacity to do the behavior. Capability deals with knowledge, psychological skills, and physical skills. **Opportunity** is defined as all the factors that lie outside the individual that make the behavior possible or prompt it.

GOALS AND SYSTEMS

Ecological models of behavior change identify several levels of influence on behavior.[3] These include individual factors, social network factors, institutional factors, community, and environmental factors, and even government policy. Changing individual factors is much easier than changing policy level factors. For example, it is a lot easier to plan to go for a walk than it is to convince your local government to build a park.

I like to focus more on what you can control and change with relative ease. We work with three levels influence in your system: individual, relationship, and structural. Individual refers to all the things going on in your head, it's cognitive factors. Relationship describes your social network, and structural describes your home, work, and neighborhood. All of these levels of influence effect motivation, opportunity, and capability. You can think of these levels as either barrier producing or goal facilitating. They either help you or hurt you.

A key principle of these ecological models is that change is easier when interventions focus on all levels of influence. I encourage you to do the same. Your system describes how the individual, relationship, and structural levels influence your motivation, opportunity, or capability.

YOUR SYSTEM			
	Motivation	Opportunity	Capability
Individual			
Relationship			
Structural			

If you are like most people, you do not struggle seeing the value in changing your behavior. Not acting, or not acting consistently, puts you in a state of **ambivalence**. Ambivalence is characterized by wanting to change and at the same time, not wanting to change. If you are stuck in ambivalence, it is not your fault. It is your system that is working against you, preventing you from executing your plan. To stay consistent and make a long-term change, we need to make your system work for you.

Changing behavior can be a fundamentally unstable and unsteady process; you should expect a fair share of lapses in self-control and relapses into old behaviors. When this happens do not fret, you are not a failure. Far from it. Rather, you have gained valuable information. You can find out where the weak link in your system is. Just like an engineer, you find out what is wrong and fix it. You will always ask yourself, why didn't I do the behavior and what influenced that?

An Example

During the COVID-19 pandemic, I was staying at my aunt's house in Vermont whenever I could. It is three hours away from Boston, secluded, and happens to be one of my favorite places. Step onto the road, take a right and you have got a mile and a half uphill run.

I went on this run each time I visited, and there were still times when I needed to walk. I'd think, "How great would it be if I could run this hill without walking?" That is my goal.

Let's examine my system to see what is in place and what could be in place to help.

	Motivation	Opportunity	Capability
Individual	This is an interesting and achievable challenge that I will take pride in I could make a playlist of my top 10 most motivating songs	Make an action plan: After I want a break from writing in the morning, I will run	I need to enhance my aerobic capacity and muscular endurance. I need to examine how many times I stop now and then try to cut back by one for each subsequent run. I am confident I can accomplish this goal
Relationship	I can tell my friends about my goal, so I am held accountable	I can bring friends or family to the house and ask them to remind me to do the run if I have not done it by 9:00am	I can ask someone who is in better shape than me to run as well.
Structural	The scenery for this run is beautiful which makes it enjoyable	The hill exists so the opportunity is there	The physical run is tough, but it is not a huge stretch from my current capabilities

After filling in my system, it is evident that this goal can work. At the structural level, everything is in place for success. At the relationship level, I could recruit help in each category. At the individual level,

I can do things to enhance my motivation during the run, I can set up an action plan as a prompt, and I can set weekly goals to ensure I am progressing. Now let's examine what could work against me.

	Motivation	Opportunity	Capability
Individual	Whenever I start running my brain tells me to stop. I don't override this thought and stop running	I fail to plan when to do the run	I don't stick with the progression plan. When the time comes to do the run, I am not in good enough shape
Relationship	N/A	None of my friends come to the house	Even if my friends are there, they do not want to do the run with me
Structural	It could be a rainy day	I live three hours away so there may be times when I cannot come	N/A

When running gets tough, my brain has the tendency to tell me to stop. To overcome this tendency, I would need to plan to recognize and override that voice in my head. It is also entirely possible that I do not plan when I am going to run, and the day goes by. If I do not train enough, even if I want to achieve this goal, my capabilities will not be there. Your best intentions only explain a percent of behavior. Good intentions cannot overcome a bad system. The goal is to set up a system that works for your goals, not against them.

You have your aspiration; you have set your three-month goal and weekly goals. Now it is time to execute the plan. We want to address the sources of influence so anything that was working against you begins to work for you. Let's break down the system into individual behavior change techniques to help you act on your plans.

THE SYSTEM THAT WORKS FOR YOU

Behavior is dichotomous. Either it happens or it does not.

The approach I am recommending is based on your system. It includes determinants of behavior at three levels of influence and states that these determinants and sources of influence contribute to behavior. The message is this: if we know what influences us, we can design an intervention to maximize our chances of success.

Behavior change techniques are essentially inputs used to change the determinants of behavior. There has been extensive research on the use of behavior change techniques in a variety of areas. I will provide you with some of my favorite techniques to either enhance motivation, opportunity, or capabilities, OR reduce the need for it.

Before You Continue

Tailored interventions work much better than generic ones. Tailored interventions take the individual into account. My writing below is a bit of a shotgun approach. Something in here should work for everyone. I would recommend you read it all, but once you start trying to change something, examine what is making adherence challenging. Once you have determined where the issue is, skip to the applicable section and try one of the techniques. From here, we will cover motivation, opportunity, and capability enhancing behavior change techniques.

ENHANCE OR REDUCE THE NEED FOR MOTIVATION WITH CHANGES AT THE INDIVIDUAL LEVEL

Motivation has two subcomponents, the *reflective side,* and the *automatic side.* Reflective processes involve planning to act on your intentions as well as the evaluation of the behavior as good or bad. It is analytical. Automatic processing involves emotional reactions and desires. One of the best books describing this is *Switch*[4] by Dan and Chip Heath. In their book they paint the picture of an elephant and a rider. The rider is the reflective process of motivation, and the elephant is the automatic side. If the rider wants to go in one direction and the elephant in the other, the elephant is going to win.

Comparing your rational brain to this emotional animal or beast is nothing new. The fight between our conscious good intentions and our impulses is something we can all relate to. In his 2011 paper,[5] Dr. Malte Friese compares the reflective side once again to a rider and the automatic side to a horse. He writes:

Picture a rider sitting on the back of his horse on a great plain. The rider seems to be somewhat aimless, orienting himself on where to go next when the horse suddenly starts bolting, taking off in a direction the rider never intended to go. While the horse is getting wild and wilder the rider can hardly keep himself on the horse's back. For future horse rides, at least three things would be helpful for the rider: **First, a better idea on where to go;** *second,* **better strength to control the horse,** *and third,* **a tamed horse** *that doesn't willfully take off to anywhere it catches a glimpse of something interesting.*

When I read this, I think of three things. First, **we need direction to implement the behaviors** we want to do. Up until now, much of this book has been about that. Next, it is beneficial to **increase our strength to go against the counterproductive impulses**. Last, Friese recommends taming that side of you.

In this section we focus on reducing the need for motivation, improving your reflective motivation, and then getting automatic motivation to work for you instead of against you.

Automate the Behavior

Imagine this: you are at Six Flags theme park staring up at the 221-foot ride, the Superman. This looks steep you say to yourself, 72-degree angle steep. You are frightened but make it through the line. You sit in your seat and are strapped in. At this point there is not turning back. You ae just along for the ride now.

When I think about automating behavior, I think, how can we just be along for the ride now? The outcome we want is already predetermined, so we cannot escape the path of action. Through personal training, people pay me to automate their behavior. Of course, I do more than this, but people pay me, they have an appointment, and they do what I have planned for the day. They are along for the ride. I recently used the Peloton in my apartment complex. As soon as I sat down, I was literally "along for the ride." For most people, hiring a permanent trainer is not in the cards. We need other options for automating our behaviors.

Imagine that you are trying to be healthier, but you go out with your friends on Friday and Saturday. Despite your good intentions you often drink double what you wanted to. You wake up in the morning, feel awful and see the pizza crust you missed next to the floor on the couch, evidence of the pepperoni and cheese massacre that happened at 3:00am last night. You certainly do not exercise that day.

What can you do? What if when you got to the bar you slipped the bartender 20 dollars and asked to give you soda water every time you came to the bar. You still look like you are drinking but you are not, and it is not even in your control anymore. You have outsourced the behavior to someone else.

Often, the hardest part about getting to the gym is getting there. In my health behavior change class we talk about automating behavior. Here was an example we came up with; Uber has a feature where you can schedule a ride for a given time. The night before, when you feel motivated to go to the gym, schedule a ride to take you there. If you get in the car and the car takes you to the gym you are not going to turn around. We will get into this later, but mobilizing social support is a sure-fire way to automate your behavior when your motivation is low.

How do you automate your behavior? Find the first step that once started will get the wheels in motion. Break down your behavior into the steps that need to happen for you to do it. Right now, I have this small exercise room in my guest room. I know that if I go into the room, I will exercise. My first step is to make sure I go into the room (dressed appropriately of course). Making an appointment for an exercise class is another surefire way to ensure that you go with a monetary commitment that is far less than that of a personal trainer. Apps that allow you to book classes online include: Mindbody, WellnessLiving, StudioBookings, Glofox, Fitli, and fitDEGREE.

De-Automate Behavior with Stopping Points

How do you de-automate an unwanted behavior? I was recently speaking to a client who wanted to be more mindful of his eating. He has an application on his phone that makes it easy to order any food he wants. I talked to him about designing **stopping points.** Behavior is due to a sequence of events.

For this client, it would look like this:

- Urge

- Pull out phone

- Open application

- Place order

- Receive order

- Eat food

Where is the most useless stopping point? Trying to get yourself to stop after you open the application. Where is the best stopping point? Likely if you could get the urge to never happen. That part is a lot harder though. What about opening up the application? If he deletes the application and makes redownloading it contingent upon entering a password that would make the behavior more challenging. Perhaps it would be a sufficient stopping point to gain control over those impulses.

TEMPTATION BUNDLING

Before she was a professor at the Wharton School of Business with the University of Pennsylvania, Katherine Milkman was a graduate student at Harvard. She had gone to the gym frequently during her undergraduate career but now lacked the energy. In an interview with NPR, she said at the end of the day she just wanted to "watch TV or read Harry Potter".[6] Milkman found a way to pair what she wanted to do (indulge in Harry Potter) with what she needed to do (exercise).

How can we take something we may be on the fence about and hop onto the side of action?

Let's say that you lacked motivation. We can make the outcome more attractive. One way to do this is to link something you want to do with something you know you should do. I have several podcasts that I like including "Up First" with NPR, "The Daily" with the *New York Times*, and "Scared to Death" a comedy horror podcast.

I also know that every night I need to take Scout for a walk. If I have low motivation and thought a short walk would suffice, I could link one of these podcasts to the behavior. Up First would get me half a mile, The Daily would get me to go for a mile and Scared to Death could be up to 3 miles if I wanted it to be. Because these podcasts are interesting, I am not tempted to stop[6] early since this would mean I would be done listening.

This is exactly the strategy that Milkman used. She loved fantasy books and was only allowed to listen to them while she was in the gym. She paired something she had to do with something she wanted to do, and it worked! Milkman calls this technique temptation bundling. You may also want to link contingent rewards with the behavior you know you should be doing. My class laughed at me when I told them that I would link running with Scout two times per week for four weeks with getting a pedicure. (Yes, men get pedicures, too.)

STIMULUS CONTROL

In his 2014 paper,[7] in Preventative Medicine, Dr. Mark Bouton discusses why it is so challenging to maintain behavior change. He says that even after a bad habit has been extinguished, we cannot ignore the intertwined relationship with context, cues, and responses. He says:

When the trigger cue is returned to the context where the behavior was learned, when the context where the behavior was extinguished is merely changed, or when the context is associated with the reinforcer again, the cue can trigger responding in our old ways again.

Stimulus control describes situations in which a behavior is triggered by a stimulus/cue. Habits form when behaviors are repeated in the same contexts if the behavior provides a reward. Once repeated behaviors that generate a reward are reinforced, we experience a craving when we are cued to do the behavior.

Stimuli, or the cue, fit into one of six categories, **location, time, emotional state, antecedents, visibility/proximity,** and **other people.** Location falls into the structural level of our system and other people fall into the relational level. Emotions that trigger behavior (i.e., stress eating) are less likely to be changed. For example, you are going to get stressed, you are going to get sad, and I do not think we should shy away from negative emotions or even try to avoid them. I think we should accept them. In this case, I would prefer to have someone identify what needs are not being met that caused a negative emotion and then identify an alternative behavior that can satisfy those needs. So, we have time, antecedents, and visibility/proximity as modifiable triggers.

Time

In my lectures, if I fail to be interesting, or even if I am interesting, my students begin to pack up about three minutes before the end of class. *Specific time* prompts them to pack up. I understand this. As an avid fan of nighttime eating, 10:00pm, usually around bedtime, is a prompt for me to see if there is anything tasty in the fridge. If there isn't, I will close the fridge and open it again, hoping that the magic fridge fairy dropped in a tasty treat for me. It never happens. Time, as a stimulus is not going to change. Once again, we are stuck with changing the behavior or removing behavioral options.

Antecedents

You stop at a red light, you go at a green light, you walk into the bathroom you brush your teeth, you get in the car and put on a seat belt. Preceding events, or antecedents are one of the most reliable prompts for a habit to occur. We modify antecedents as stimulus control. To break a bad habit, identify the behavior you want to change. Simply observe at this point. Is your prompt to do the behavior an earlier behavior? For example, each morning on his way to work my dad told me he would stop to grab a coffee at one of the gas stations on his way in.

While gas stations may have a killer $0.99 coffee deal, they also happen to be riddled with pop tarts, packaged pastries, and candy. Even if Dad, with the best of his intentions went in to get a coffee he had unknowingly created a habit loop where stopping to get coffee triggered the urge to buy candy, Pop tarts, and pastries. The simple solution is to avoid stopping at the gas station. Make coffee at home or go through a drive through to purchase coffee instead.

Visibility/Proximity

One of my clients struggled with cell phone use at work. If he had his phone, he would spend hours browsing Reddit, Instagram, and YouTube. Prior to Covid-19, he would leave his phone at home, but now while working from home, he could not escape his phone. Wasting time on his phone would set off a cascade that would influence his ability to exercise. He would think to himself that he had wasted so much time on his phone that he should not exercise and should continue to work.

He was stuck in a cycle. He would finish a task (the cue), feel the urge to look at his cell phone (urge), and take out his phone (routine). We talked about what he has tried so far. He had put it in his desk at work. That didn't work. He tried throwing the phone on his bed. That didn't work.

The reason why these techniques did not work was because he only addressed visibility or proximity, not both. What he decided to do was to give his phone to his wife during the day. Out of sight out of mind. He expressed that while he felt the strong urge to use his phone, he also knew he could not go and ask his wife to use his phone to look at Instagram during work hours.

HABIT FORMATION WITH REINFORCEMENT

Reinforcement is going to be a factor in determining whether a stimulus leads to a behavior that we approach or a behavior that we avoid. If a behavior is associated with a positive outcome, we approach it. If it is connected to a negative one, we avoid it. Stanford professor and Author BJ Fogg encourages people to start tiny. He says,[8] take any new habit you want to form and scale it back. Pick a behavior that is so easy to do. Rob yourself of any excuse. When you have found out what you want to do, you are going to use a technique you will learn more about soon, an implementation intention. Link the behavior you want to do with something you are already doing. Once you have done the behavior, reinforce it with a positive outcome. You need to feel successful!

Make sure that you repeat the behavior in the same context. That is, if you decide to do yoga after your first cup of coffee in the morning, make sure you repeat it in the same sequence and under the same circumstances. Aside from finding behaviors that provide intrinsic rewards, think about how you can feel good when you are done. How would you like to celebrate a job well done?

DECISIONAL BALANCE

Decisional balance involves weighing the pros and cons of staying the same and the pros and cons of making a change.

If you feel stuck, it can be helpful to write out all the pros and cons of changing and the pros and cons of staying the same. To recognize that the pros of changing outweigh the cons and that the cons of staying the same outweigh the pros can be a powerful tool. The only issue with this technique is that some people may identify more reasons not to change.

Imagine Future Outcomes (10/10/10)

Psychological distance describes the distance between your present self and your future self. When we think about what tomorrow will look like, we can easily make a prediction. The immediate future looks a lot like the present. Consequences or benefits are in the future. This makes the outcome, whether positive or negative, an abstraction.

It is hard to wrap our mind around a heart attack 30 years from now, or a 10% reduction in body fat three years from now, but let's try. The point of this exercise is to bring the future to the present. If this technique elicits some form of emotion driven motivation it is important to supplement it with a plan.

Susan Welch[9] calls her technique, 10/10/10. With this technique you imagine that you made a decision. Maybe it is to pick up exercising. How will your life be different after you made this decision 10 minutes from now? How about 10 months from now? What about 10 years from now. I think the 10/10/10 rule can also work well for tough one-time decisions. Imagine that you are concerned about going to the gym. You feel that you will embarrass yourself. For all intents and purposes let's say you do something that is embarrassing. How will you feel 10 minutes after this happened?

Likely still embarrassed. How about 10 months from now? This will probably be a fleeting memory. What about 10 years from now. You will not remember it happened.

Widen the Options

When we think of behavior in terms of **this or that,** we fail to examine the multitude of choices we have. If I do not exercise at 3:00pm, I will not have time to do it today. If I want to lose weight, I cannot have pizza anymore. If I go for a walk, I will not have time to spend with my family.

Change can seem unappealing if you immediately go to black and white decision-making. If losing weight means giving up pizza, I am out! If I spend an hour exercising every day my wife will kill me! We need to stop thinking in terms of only having two options and accept the plethora of choices at hand.

Write down a behavior you have wanted to do, and then write down the barriers. Why might this behavior be unappealing? What would demotivate you? Then examine your options. In terms of ways to exercise, do not get attached to one method. If you do not have time to go to the gym, that does not mean you cannot go for a walk, do a body weight circuit at home, follow a yoga video, or go for a run. Do not be so quick to latch onto the first behavioral option that pops into your head. If you think that the path to fitness means buying a fancy piece of home exercise equipment, joining a gym, or joining boot camp style classes you need to widen your view on the available options.

COUNTER CONDITIONING

It is common practice to replace unhealthy behaviors with healthier options. This is called counterconditioning. Counterconditioning hijacks the response part of the habit loop. You change your routine in response to a stimulus. Specifically, choose a stimulus that would elicit a negative response and replace it with a positive response. For example, does being bored make you want to eat? Does being stressed make you want to drink? Does being anxious keep you out of the gym?

Remember that even the behaviors we want to change have immediate beneficial outcomes. Drinking can ease stress, eating can ease boredom, avoidance of situations can reduce anxiety. Think about the situations leading up to the behavior you want to change. What are the antecedents? Next, think about why it happens, what need is the problematic behavior fulfilling. Then think about what you can do instead. See if the urge to do the problematic behavior has stayed the same, gotten stronger, or reduced. If your urge is reduced stick with the behavioral alternative you chose.

BEHAVIOR-VALUE CONGRUENCE

I am assuming that some of your default decisions are not the ones you want to make. Deliberate, non-default decisions take effort. These types of choices are more likely to be made if they are linked to goals that are based on deeply felt values.

Let me tell you a story from the book, *Motivational Interviewing*,[10] about a father who quit smoking. He had drove to pick his kids up at the city library. A thunderstorm greeted him as he pulled up. The father searched his pockets to find cigarettes and realized he was out. He looked up at the library and saw his children walking out into the rain but continued to search for a parking spot where he could run into a store, buy cigarettes, and be back before his kids got seriously wet.

This view of himself as the kind of father who would let his kids get drenched by a thunderstorm caused him to immediately quit. When our behaviors come into conflict with our values it is our behaviors that change, not our values. Think about what you want to change. Where does the struggle lie? What things make it hard to change? What are your default behaviors that make it tough to get out of your own way?

Do you find yourself missing workouts, eating junk food, or otherwise coping with your problems in nonproductive ways? Most people I speak with want one of three things, they want more confidence, they want more balance, and they want more control. What do you want? When I type this question, I write it with a sense of genuine interest; how do your problematic behaviors fit in with your aspirations? How does eating junk food when you feel stressed fit in with your aspiration of having more control over behavior? How does missing workouts or being sedentary for too long fit with managing your diabetes?

Make It Autonomous

Autonomous motivation happens when you do a behavior because you want to do it. This could mean you find the behavior fun; consistent with your identity, or you value the outcome of the behavior. If a behavior is enjoyable, part of your identity, and/or if you value the outcome you are going to persist in the behavior. The other form of motivation, controlled motivation relates to external contingencies, specifically, reward and punishment. People that act for approval from others, for avoidance of shame, and for ego-enhancements also have controlled motivation. People with controlled motivation do not self-endorse their behavior, rather they feel pressure to do the behavior. Autonomous motivation leads to superior long-term perseverance toward health behaviors.

In November of 2017, I was home for Thanksgiving break. One of the creators of Self-Determination theory, Edward Deci worked about an hour away from me. I had emailed him a month back to see if I could meet him when I was home. Surprisingly (surprisingly because he is a big deal) he responded and said yes. We spoke for about an hour. I talked to him about his concept of autonomous motivation. How do we become autonomously motivated? Dr. Deci told me we need to have our psychological needs met. Our psychological needs include autonomy, competency, and related-ness. Autonomy refers to the need to feel control over the behavior they are doing. Competency refers to building mastery around the behavior. Relatedness, or connection, refers to needing to feel cared for or cared about.

This concept overlaps with confidence and capabilities and with various sources of influence. It also connects with the last point of having a positive aspiration for your health. Having an intrinsic aspiration such as personal development linked to the health behavior can serve as a reminder for why you are doing what you are doing when things become challenging.

DON'T BREAK THE CHAIN

As kids, my brother and I would make Christmas chains. These were loops of paper linked together. Starting in December, every morning we would go downstairs and take one loop off. Another day closer to Christmas, we were excited to go downstairs and rip that paper off because it meant another day closer to presents.

Author James Clear discusses the "don't break the chain"[11] strategy for making habits stick. The goal is to pick a behavior you want to do, and each time you do it, mark an X on a calendar.

Here is what I recommend. Pick one behavior you want to do every day. Something that gets you moving or some low hanging fruit for nutrition. For example, maybe that is a 20 minute walk every day. Maybe it means having vegetables with every dinner. For this, your goal is to never break the chain.

You should also try something challenging. For example, jogging, lifting, making a home cooked healthy meal. For this, make it your goal to never miss two days in a row.

CLOSE THE CIRCLE

This technique is related to not breaking the chain. I was speaking with one of my clients about why he loves his Apple Watch. With the Apple Watch, you can set a goal and when you complete it you watch the rings on the screen close in. As you get closer to your goal you get closer to seeing the rings close. The fact that they are almost closed can be a motivating force for extra physical activity. You close the rings, the screen lights up, it says goal achieved, and you feel good. My client said it is so rare in life that you actually get to finish or accomplish anything. Most things are ongoing tasks. Work is an ongoing task; fitness is an ongoing task. Finishing something is rewarding. One thing this client and I decided he would do to experience task completion and to mimic the apple watch rings was to get two jars and 30 marbles. Every day that he completed two health related tasks he would move a marble over to the "good jar." If he did not do two tasks, he would have to move a marble from the "good jar" to the "bad jar." This served as a visible representation of task completion.

ENHANCE OR REDUCE THE NEED FOR MOTIVATION WITH CHANGES AT THE RELATIONSHIP LEVEL

Justin's Law of Social Sabotage

In 1686, Sir Isaac Newton introduced his three laws of motion in *Principia Mathematica Philosophiae Naturalis*. Newton's Third Law states that for every action in nature, there is an equal and opposite reaction.

I am often asked what to do when attempts to be healthy are sabotaged by significant others. Why, when we try to be healthy do friends, family, and spouses consciously or unconsciously try to stop us. Often, their responses are not malicious. Your desire to change can cause an emotional reaction. Reactions and the extent to which someone responds to your behaviors is a reflection of what that means to them within the context their lives.

Let's say you have a significant other get upset with you for something you did. You put your jacket on the chair, not the coat hanger. Their reaction should be a 1 out of 10 but instead it's a 5 out of 10. Something else caused the elevated reaction. Perhaps it was the fact that they have asked you to not do this. Maybe they have had a really tough day at work. Maybe they had a fight with a family member. Either way, something else caused the elevated reaction.

If you eat vegetables and that makes someone in your social circle upset, this is because something else is happening on their side of the equation. Here is my law of social sabotage: "**A behavior and its meaning to the other person is proportional to the reaction.**"

If, for whatever reason, I keyed someone's car right in front of them, they should flip out. They should have an elevated reaction. They would yell at me, call the cops, or punch me in the face. Their reaction will be based on what it means to in the context of my bad behavior. Exercising should mean nothing to someone else. If someone makes snide remarks about you exercising it is because it makes them feel a certain way. Maybe it makes them feel insecure that they are not exercising.

What to do? Be clear in your conversation with that person. Tell them how their behaviors influence you. Tell them that their reactions to you trying to improve yourself hurt, and just as importantly, tell them that you would like to listen and understand why they are doing what they are doing. Then, actually do what you said you would do, listen! It is not your behavior that is the problem if you are trying to be healthy, it is how your behavior is making someone else feel.

LEARN TO RESIST SOCIAL PRESSURE

You are at a family gathering, you have been trying with Herculean effort to be healthy the last few weeks. Out comes the snacks. It is those dates filled with peanut butter that you love so much and what is that to the left? More dates, but filled with cream cheese and then wrapped around it is a piece of bacon? You might white knuckle it for the first round, but then your uncle asks you if you want a beer, and then so does your cousin. You say no, they say come on, you say no, they persist, but you still survive. Then it's cake time. You try to stay away, on the outskirts of the party, that seemed like the safest option. Cake doesn't have legs, it can't travel. Or can it...

Your aunt starts making the rounds with the slices. She puts a plate in front of you. It's one of those corner pieces, the kind where all the frosting is. You say no, but she insists. You cave! And when the cake it done you polish off the remainder of the plate of dates.

Does this situation sound familiar? You are trying to be good only to be unwittingly sabotaged by friends and family? What can we do, aside from avoiding people, to resist social pressure? It is hard enough to resist junk food without people trying to shove it down your throat. So, you need some tools. What if you could elicit an automatic response from your would-be saboteur to simply leave you alone?

In a 1989 study, Harvard Psychologist Ellen Langer[12] sought to study compliance. Specifically, would someone comply to a favor if we gave them a reason why? In her study she wanted to see if people would allow her participants to budge them in line if they gave a reason for why they needed to budge. When people asked to cut to make copies on a xerox machine they were allowed to do so 60% of the time. But when they gave a reason why they needed to cut they were allowed to cut 93% of the time! This was even when the reason did not add any new information. For example, one group just said, can I cut because I need to make copies. The secret sauce was not the reason, it was simply the use of the word *because*. I was interested in testing this with one of my clients. She had a scenario that would often go down like this:

Situation 1:

Boyfriend: "Do you want a glass of wine?"

Girlfriend: "No, thank you."

Boyfriend: "Are you sure you don't want any?"

Girlfriend: "Yes."

Boyfriend: "Here just have a little." (At this point, boyfriend pours half a glass of wine).

I told her that the next time he asks you if you want alcohol to simply say "no thank you because" and then give literally any reason.

Here is how situation 2 went:

Situation 2:

Boyfriend: "Do you want a glass of wine?"

Girlfriend: "No, thank you, I'm good because I'm actually feeling a little dehydrated."

Boyfriend: "Let me get you a glass of water!"

Using the "Because…" strategy effectively takes away any chance for the other party to resist.

ELICIT SUPPORT FROM FRIENDS

My friend Jo has run a couple of marathons including the Boston Marathon. Every once and a while, I would join her on a leg of her run. Running three miles was fine, but I was not the only running buddy she had on a given day. As a matter of fact, she was picking people up and dropping them off as she went along. One person would run five miles, another three, then maybe one more person would finish out the run with her. This way, she was always held accountable in her training.

Social support is a powerful tool. It is a way to outsource the need for motivation. When it is warm in Boston, I am guaranteed to run a 5k at least one time per week because I set up a 5k club with the gym I work at. Every Monday at around 5:30, a group of us would meet up outside the gym and then run across the Charles River to MIT and back to the gym on Bolyston Street.

The enabling hypothesis[13] states that receiving social support may help a person self-regulate their behavior by enabling them to master the challenge at hand. Social support is such a powerful tool because it can enhance your sense of self-efficacy and it is a perfect way to outsource self-regulation. Setting a goal with a partner may also keep you motivated and on track for your goal.

OBSERVE DESCRIPTIVE AND SUBJECTIVE NORMS

In 2007, Nicholas Christakis and James Fowler published a paper[14] that shed insight into the effect of the social environment on obesity. If a close friend, a spouse, or sibling becomes obese, the odds that you will become obese will increase.

I found social influencing fascinating. My master's thesis focused on what is called descriptive norms. **Descriptive norms** refer to the perception of what most people do. On the other hand, **injunctive norms** refer to norms that characterize the perception approval or disapproval of a behavior. Descriptive norms have a powerful unconscious pull on our own behavior. If a large group of people are staring up at a building when you pass by, you will also look up. Social psychological researcher and author, Robert Cialdini, writes[15] that descriptive norms motivate by providing evidence as to what will likely be effective and adaptive action:

If everyone is doing or thinking or believing it, it must be a sensible thing to do or think or believe.

We see this in our social interactions. When people eat in groups[16] they tend to eat more than if they were alone. People model the eating behavior of who they are with. If the person you are with consumes more than you normally would, you will eat more than if they were a light eater.

Imagine that you are with an immediate social network, specifically, your three closest friends. Friend 1 is very healthy, but friends 2 and 3 have unhealthy habits. First be aware of the situations where you behave differently than you would like to in the presence of friend 2 and friend 3. Maybe friend 2 and 3 are sedentary. Maybe friend 2 and 3 drink too much or always have unhealthy food around. You can be more mindful of the circumstances that you encounter when you are with them and mentally prepare for interactions. You can also try to spend more time within the social circle that friend 1 inhabits. Maybe she walks daily. Can you join them for something? If you do this, odds are you will get acquainted with their social circle.

Whether fortunate or unfortunate, once you start to buy into a healthy lifestyle you often outgrow the people that do not align with your vision of health. For a lack of a better word, we might outgrow our relationships with people that hold us back.

COMMITMENT DEVICES

One of my clients desperately wanted to reduce his phone use. It was a time suck. It made him unproductive at work and interfered with his plans to exercise. He tried giving it to his wife during the day but was very inconsistent with that. He talked about getting a burner phone that had no internet service, but that was a bit extreme. Nothing was working. So, we tried…punishment.

As a note, I don't think this strategy works long term. To be clear the punishment was financial not physical. This client decided that he would put down a monetary incentive that would be painful enough to lose. He decided to pick a political candidate to donate to that he believed would not win (but wouldn't mind if this candidate did). If he looked at his phone, he would need to donate $100.00 dollars to this candidate's campaign. I have a daily reminder to him to see how the day went. If he looked at his phone, he owes me a screen shot of the donation. Another one of my clients knew that going out and drinking was interfering with her weight loss. It was a tough habit to kick. She ended up sending one of her friends $300.00 which could only be returned if she did not go out that night.

Now, if you really want to stop doing something, or start doing something, and you are an honest person who is loss averse, find a cause you're not keen on donating to. Pick a price that will not break the bank, but you won't be thrilled about losing.

Make the behavior crystal clear:

- I will walk three times this week for 20 minutes.

- I will eat vegetables every day.

- I will lift weights twice per week for 20 minutes.

Put down a monetary amount that you are comfortable but not happy about losing. Find a friend to check in with daily or weekly. If you break your contract, you need to up the ante.

ENHANCE OR REDUCE THE NEED FOR MOTIVATION WITH CHANGES AT THE STRUCTURAL LEVEL

World renowned researcher Jim Sallis writes[17] "diet and physical activity interventions that build knowledge, motivation, and behavior change skills in individuals without changing the environments in which they live are unlikely to be effective. Similarly, merely changing the physical activity or the food environment may not be sufficient for a substantial change in behavior."

If we do not change our structural environment, we will need to expend more and more willpower and motivation to do healthy things and more and more willpower and motivation to resist unhealthy things. Why not create the path of least resistance by making structural changes to our environment?

I am not an avid runner in Boston. As I noted earlier, I formed by own 5k club as a commitment to make sure I ran three miles at least one time per week, but when I find myself in Vermont, it is so much easier. The scenery is beautiful, I'm always the only one on the road, and it is hard to beat running beside a lake.

The structural level of influence is interesting to me. You can easily change your home environment, maybe less easily change your work environment, but you certainly cannot will a park, trail, or beautiful lake into existence. You can improve your home environment to make healthy choices easier, but in terms of the environment that promotes healthier lifestyle choices we really need to examine our options. We need to look for what might have been right in front of us the whole time.

Examine Available Options

I lived in Boston for two years before I used a bike share program. After the end of one of my 5k runs we would all hang out for a little bit at the bar next to the gym. My roommate and I had two options to get home. The first was to call an Uber and the second was to take the train. To commute with the train, we would need to walk half a mile to the T stop, ride the T to Harvard Square and then walk a mile and a half to our place or wait for the bus to take us there.

No appealing commuting option existed for me, but it was a nice night, and we noticed the Blue Bikes, Boston's bike share program. Blue Bikes are everywhere in Boston, Cambridge, and Somerville. You would be hard pressed to walk a quarter mile without seeing one (they have 1,800 bikes). So, we took the bike and it ended up being a lovely ride along the Charles River and over the bridge towards MIT. It was much more pleasurable than being crammed onto the train. I bought a year pass which was something like $99.00 and almost always biked when it was an option.

According to Wikipedia, 58 cities have bike share programs. In Boston, active transportation director, Stefanie Seskin's[18] job is to make walking and biking a more attractive option. Not only was the opportunity to ride a bike expanded through a partnership with Blue Cross Blue Shield, but bike lanes are all over the city of Boston which makes riding safer. These bikes are accessible, safe, and affordable.

My opportunity to utilize active transportation methods (bike or walk) is much different than my parents who live in the suburbs. They cannot bike or walk to work. The bike sharing program is not there and the distance is too far. I don't need to be exceptionally motivated to ride a bike either. The commute time on the T in Boston is actually greater than riding the bike and the T is not exceptionally appealing. The bike is a no brainer when the weather is nice.

Find Aesthetically Pleasing Choices

Your opportunity to do physical activity will come in four categories,[19] occupational, household, transport, and leisure-time. While no consistent evidence exists, leisure time activity is related to transportation environment, this includes pavement and safety, aesthetics (greenness and attractiveness), and to proximity to recreational areas. Take the chart below and think about what transportation options you have where you can include more physical activity. Maybe that means walking to the store, work, or to a friend's house. Next, where are some areas that you find aesthetically pleasing? Is it a park? A lake? Where can you go where you will enjoy yourself? Then examine if it is close enough for you to use without it being hassle.

	Option 1	Option 2	Option 3	Option 4
Transportation				
Aesthetically pleasing				
Close				

Here is an example: I wrote down transportation options and then aesthetically pleasing options then determined if these aesthetically pleasing options are close and therefore viable.

	Option 1	Option 2	Option 3	Option 4
Transportation	Ride blue bikes to work	Walk from Park Street to work rather than switch lines	Jog home from Harvard Square rather than waiting for the bus	Walk to the grocery store (1 mile away) when we don't need a lot
Aesthetically pleasing	Run around Fresh Pond Park	Run club on the Charles River	Hill run in Vermont	Run to Carson Beach with Scout
Close	X	X		X

Examine your environment, whether through an internet search or a mental search to see what you can come up with to add extra physical activity into your life.

Nudge Yourself

The other day I was shopping, and I saw the cookies that my girlfriend likes. Being the best boyfriend that I am, I bought those cookies. She was so excited to come home to see them on her nightstand. She bites into a cookie, devouring it in seconds. She reaches for the next one and sends it to meet its maker. She reaches for a third and looks over at me:

"Want a cookie?" she asks.

"I'm all set."

Her eyes get bigger, "You don't want one cookie?"

"Okay, one."

One turned into two. It was counterproductive. I realize I was the architect of my own destruction in that moment. To be clear, a cookie is not bad. Eating multiple cookies just does not match with my health goals, but I ate it, and I ate it because the choice was salient. Many of our unhealthy decisions are mindless in nature. The goal of adjusting your environment is to automatically nudge yourself to make a healthier choice.

A nudge[20] is "any aspect of the choice architecture that alters people's behavior without forbidding any options or significantly changing their economic incentives." Nudging puts you in a position where you will not have to use willpower to overcome temptation. A good self-nudge is about avoiding the cause of temptation, so in that sense it is a lot like stimulus control. In an interview with Today, Tara Swart from MIT says to start with small tweaks to nudge yourself in the right direction. "You can take on bigger challenges as you develop the skill of self-nudging".[21] The article in *Today* recommends changing position and accessibility as ways to nudge healthier decisions.

Positioning

Positioning is as simple as making the healthy choice visible and the less healthy choice invisible. Visibility enhancement[22] is one-way grocery stores and restaurants have nudged people to make healthier decisions. This is a cognitive strategy that enhances the visibility of the healthy option by placing it at eye level. Unhealthy options get placed on bottom shelves or in the middle of restaurant menus. The goal is to draw attention to the healthier option. If restaurants and grocery stores can do this, so can you!

Accessibility

Availability of, and proximity to recreational areas is associated with physical activity. Having access to healthy options can have a profound impact on whether or not you are physically active. If the closest gym to you is 50 miles away, there is no way that you are going to make a 100-mile round trip to exercise. The thought will not even cross your mind. Similarly, if there are pastries on your kitchen table and fruit in your garage fridge, we can predict with relative ease what you will choose. The less accessible the healthy choice is, the more motivation you need to overcome this barrier. The more accessible an unhealthy choice is, the more motivation you need to resist it. For example, in one study,[23] researchers found that office secretaries ate 3 more Hersey kisses when candy was visible compared to not visible. The only difference in conditions was that one jar was clear and the other was opaque!

Here is what I encourage. You must find what you can do and what you want to do. Unfortunately, if you do not live by a park, you cannot go for a walk in the park. If you do not own a bike you cannot go for a bike ride. Examine your environment and look for opportunities for physical activity. In terms of food, make your healthy choices more visible, and unhealthy choices less visible.

CREATE OPPORTUNITY WITH CHANGES AT THE INDIVIDUAL LEVEL

Form Action Plans

Goals necessitate time management and specific plans. Consider two important forms of planning when implementing goals: action planning and coping planning. Action planning describes when and where you will carry out your goals. An advanced form of action planning is called habit stacking. Habit stacking is when you pair a current habit with a new habit. The old habit serves as the trigger for the new habit. For example, my morning routine looks like this:

1. Wake up

2. Turn on coffee

3. Grab coffee

4. Check emails

I wanted to start running with Scout in the morning. My action plan looked like this: "If I do not have a client at 7:00am I will take Scout out for a run." I stacked this habit to occur right after I turned the coffee on.

Make Coping Plans

Good intentions do not guarantee actions. In fact, intentions only predict a moderate amount of actual behavior. Having good intentions is not enough. Making an action plan to prompt you to do something is a good start, but if you really want to close that gap between your good intentions and your behavior there needs to be something else.

Coping plans are a barrier focused self-regulation strategy. Self-regulation describes attempts to change habitual or automatic responses to stimulus or cues. When we use self-regulation strategies, we act on our intentions. Self-regulation failure can happen in several situations; when we are stressed, when we lose focus, when we are in social situations, or when we act on our habits rather than intentions.

Essentially, everything is all good until it is not. This whole chapter is about how good intentions cannot overcome a bad system. Realistically, there is no such thing as a perfect system. We will run into temptations. Certain situations may derail us if we do not have a plan in place. Coping planning[24] can help you overcome barriers by identify risky situations and making plans to deal with these situations is the proper response to the disruptive prompt. I ask all my clients this question when they tell me that they want to do something: "What could get in the way and what needs to be in place for you to be successful?"

This question works because it helps people identify barriers that may get in the way and also prompts them to identify the resources they need to respond to counterproductive prompts. A follow up question after the week has been complete is to ask yourself what you learned from your experience. Maybe you found that if you were strapped for time that you did not exercise. Your coping plan should address this specific barrier. Coping plans and action plans have a similar form.

Your coping plan should look like this: "If _____ (insert your barrier) then I will _____ (insert your plan)."

"If I am out to dinner then I will ask the waiter to box up half of my meal before he brings it out."

"If I am out to dinner then I will move the bread outside of my arms reach."

"If I am going out to dinner then I will pre decide a healthy meal by looking at the online menus first."

The combination of action planning, habit stacking, and coping planning can help to ensure that process goals are acted on.

Create a Behavioral Check List

On August 16, 1987, Northwest Airlines Flight 255 crashed, killing all but one passenger and two people on the ground. The National Transportation Safety Board concluded that the airline training and checking programs did not promote the effective use of checklist. It had already been established that checklist are valuable, indispensable tools of airline safety, but were ignored or misused.

A checklist can be a valuable behavior change tool if used correctly. One of my clients identified an issue that he had. When he felt the urge to eat unhealthy food, he would pull up his app, make the order, and voila, the food was there in 20 minutes. We identified that the problem was in the instant gratification, the quick turn over from urge to satisfaction. He wanted to interrupt that, so we designed a stopping point. He would delete the application, however, that was too small of a barrier. He decided he would try to make a checklist. This checklist would inform him if he could order the food he craved.

His checklist looked like this:

- Did I wait 20 minutes after my urge hit to see if I still wanted the food?

- Did I see if I had food in the house that I could make that would also satisfy the urge?

- Did I try having a healthy snack instead to satisfy the urge?

- Did I check my food diary to see if I have had unhealthy food recently?

I explained to him the difference between a hot and a cold situation. A hot situation occurs when you are influenced by your emotional state whereas a cool situation occurs when you are being more logical. The checklist serves as an extended stopping point to take you out of the hot situation. If you remove yourself from hot state, you will be able to make a decision based on logic. If you still want the have a burger, go for it, but try using a check list to make behavior more mindful and less impulsive.

CREATE OPPORTUNITY WITH CHANGES AT THE RELATIONSHIP LEVEL

Social support refers to aid and assistance that is received through social relationships. It is the belief that support will be there when you need it. Forms of social support include instrumental (financial assistance), appraisal (offering help), informational, and emotional. In this section, we focus on appraisal, specifically friends or family members offering to help.

Ask a Friend or Coach to Give You a Prompt

One of my clients was in a funk. He was struggling to exercise. His energy was low, his motivation was low, and he was in a rut. He wanted to get back to it, he just couldn't find his motivation. It's okay, that is why he has me. We decided on two things. The first is that we would get together and work out, and the second was that the next day he would plan on exercising at 8:30. I told him I would Facetime him at 8:30am to prompt him to exercise. I put the reminder in my calendar, invited him, and gave him a call at 8:30am. He was already on his bike.

You don't need to hire a coach to remind you to do the things you want to do. You can always ask a friend to do this for you. Let's say you want to go for a jog on Sunday. Pick a time that works for you and ask a friend to give you a call at that time. This works for a couple reasons. The first is that you just made a commitment to someone else. The second is that you have set up a dual reminder. The first failsafe is that you put it in your calendar. The second failsafe is that if you forget you will have someone to remind you. If you are struggling to get moving send a message to a good friend to ask them for help. Ask them to call you or Facetime you at the time you had planned on exercising.

CREATE OPPORTUNITY WITH CHANGES AT THE STRUCTURAL LEVEL

Decisions need to be seen as a series of choices between options. Time spent doing one thing, or decisions to do something over another thing is in part dependent on what opportunity the environment provides you. If you were equally motivated to do a healthy behavior (i.e., exercise), and an unhealth behavior (i.e., being sedentary), the easiest opportunity will prevail.

Make the Healthy Choice Easy

Logan Airport in Boston is easy. My first trip out of Logan was to Washington DC for a conference. I hoped in an Uber, got right to the gate. The way back is a little more challenging, you need to walk a little bit to the Uber pick up spot. Still, no problem. Then the rules changed. I flew into California and did a road trip which included the Grand Canyon and Las Vegas. Now Ubers had to go to a specific drop off and pick up point. My driver to Logan was kind enough to break the rules and drop us right at our terminal, but on the way back the option was not there. There were a bunch of convoluted instructed on how to get to the Uber pick up point. I walked around confused with my luggage before I gave up and went to the taxi pick up point. I clocked the price out to be $180.00 dollars per hour to ride in a taxi. It took 20 minutes to get home.

The appealing choice, a 20-minute ride for 20 dollars was not available. So, we took the less appealing choice because it was easier. Let's say you need to decide between going to the gym or playing video games. You are already on the couch, in front of the television, and the video game controller is practically in your hand. That's the easy decision. You are probably going to do that unless you are very motivated to exercise. Let's say you have left over pizza on the counter. You are probably going to eat that before you cook a healthy meal.

In 1997, Douglas Raynor, Karen Coleman, and Leonard Epstein published a study[25] that was simple and elegant. They recruited sedentary undergraduate students to study the effects of proximity on the choice to be physically active or sedentary. All participants were told to bring a pair of exercise clothes. When they arrived at the lab, they were shown several exercises and were informed that they could be physically active or engage in sedentary activities.

They were randomly assigned to one of four conditions:

1. Proximal exercise choice and proximal sedentary choice

2. Proximal exercise choice and distant sedentary choice

3. Distant exercise choice and proximal sedentary choice

4. Distant exercise choice and distant sedentary choice

Access to activities in the proximal condition were immediately accessible and activities in the distant location involved walking for five minutes. Participants in the exercise near and sedentary far conditions spent all 20 minutes engaging in exercise. However, when sedentary options were near, participants spent more time being sedentary. When we make physical activity more convenient and sedentary activity less convenient, we are more likely to be physically active.

IMPROVE CONFIDENCE AND CAPABILITIES AT THE INDIVIDUAL LEVEL

Enhance Capabilities

Over my spring break in 7th or 8th grade, my Dad took me to Golds gym. He showed me all the different machines and took me through a workout. I felt so proud of what I had accomplished. After a catching glimpse of my pumped up little 14-year-old biceps in Dad's car window I was hooked. Years later, still with my Dad at the YMCA now, I bench pressed 135 for 10 repetitions for the first time. Needless to say, I was the man.

With the gift of hindsight, my first routine was not technically challenging. I improved, but more importantly, I was excited with each level of improvement. I learned that by working a muscle and putting it under progressively more challenging circumstances, I could get stronger, I could get bigger muscles. Our psychological strengths and capabilities are like muscles. With practice, they can get stronger.

The single greatest determinant improvement is practice. You cannot expect to get better at exercising without practice. You cannot expect to get better at improving willpower without practice. You cannot expect to be better at planning without planning. You cannot will improvement into existence without action.

Enhancing capabilities is a matter of finding the appropriate amount of stress that you can handle. It is about stretching yourself to the next step without breaking. Once stretched, you attain a new normal. You adapt and then push yourself again. Examine where you are now, then find the next step. If you can walk a mile in 20 minutes, try to do it in 19. If you can do 20 push-ups, try to do 21.

Reduce Task Demand

Albert Bandura is one of the most highly cited psychological researchers of our time. He gave us the term self-efficacy, confidence in task specific abilities. In a 1969 study,[26] Bandura recruited participants to eliminate their fear of snakes. In a series of ever more threatening performance tasks, participants interacted with a 4-foot king snake. The tasks required participants to walk up to the snake in a glass cage, to look at it, to touch it, to hold the snake with a gloved hand, to hold the snake with a bare hand. This eventually led to participants holding the snake 5 inches from their face and crawling on their laps!

Participants were placed in one of four groups. One group was a no treatment control group. One group received relaxation techniques and imagined more threatening scenarios with the snake. Another group observed film where people interacted with the King snake, including draping the snake around their neck. The third group watched an experimenter with a snake and received graded increases in difficulty in interacting with the snake. Through a one-way mirror they watched the experimenter interact with the snake. Then they were asked to join the experimenter. The experimenter held the snake at the head and tail while the participants touched the snake with a gloved hand and then eventually with a bare hand. Progress to more aversive situations was based on participants apprehensiveness.

The modeling with guided practice was the most effective method for extinguishing fear arousal and improving attitudes. So where are we going with all of this? There is value in breaking down challenging tasks into their more manageable components. Let's say the end goal for exercise is to do vigorous aerobic exercise three times per week and strength training three times per week but you aren't currently doing anything. This is the same as if you asked someone who has a snake phobia to put a snake's head 5 inches from their face. You are setting them up for disaster.

It's okay to keep your eyes on the end goal. Maybe that means losing weight, running a race, lifting a certain weight, but let's break that down into its smaller components. What's the next step, not the last step? Reduce task demand to match your motivation.

Create Starter Steps

A starter step is the first step in a sequence of behaviors. For example, strength training in the gym is the result of several steps that came before it. You changed into your gym clothes, grabbed your keys, walked to your car, turned the car on and drove to the gym. Thinking of all the steps you need to take can stir up some resistance. Starter steps reduce this resistance but focus on the first thing you need to do to get the ball rolling. In this example, I might think of my starter step as getting in the car. That doesn't feel too taxing, and if I can get in the car I will go to the gym.

Reattribution Training

Reattribution training is a technique that challenges automatic thoughts and assumptions about the root cause of our behavior by considering different causes. The fundamental attribution error[27] is a cognitive error that occurs when we attribute behavior to personal dispositions rather than to situational factors. With reattribution training you reinterpret previous failures in terms of unstable characteristics (i.e., tired, stressed, environment) and successes in terms of stable attributions (hard working, determined).

Let's say that you planned on exercising three times this week but did not go once. The story you tell yourself is that you are lazy. Being lazy is a stable attribution. It's something you are telling yourself about the type of person you truly are, but what evidence in your life contradicts that assessment of yourself? Do you work a full-time job? Manage a family? Try to have a social life as well? How can you be lazy with all of these things going on? Maybe you just need to improve your time management because you were very busy (an unstable situational characteristics).

Psychological Acceptance

Internal experiences such as cravings, anxiety, sadness, or low mood can be unpleasant. You may be driven to suppress these feelings or cope with them behaviorally (i.e. drink when stressed). Avoiding the negative state may give you temporary relief to the detriment of long-term progress. Self-control requires an ability to either accept some form of distress, or to accept an immediately less pleasurable behavior for a more pleasurable one.

Physical skills for exercise and knowledge of how to make nutritious delicious meals are important components of being healthy, but it is also just as important to have the psychological skills to overcome barriers. One of those skills is acceptance. Experiential avoidance is a term that describes aversion to certain thoughts, feelings, and physical sensations even if it means causing harm in the long term.

Think about this sentence, "you don't have a problem, you have a bad solution." Having stress is not a problem; drinking, smoking, or eating to cope with it is a bad solution. Not feeling confident in your ability to exercise is not a problem but being sedentary to avoid these feelings is a bad solution.

Within my first few weeks at my PhD program, I was hit with imposter syndrome. My cohort had more basic science people, the smarty pants, and I was just this guy who was interested in behavior. They were talking about preventing diabetes with pharmacological interventions and I was talking about convincing people to move more. I did not feel worthy, I thought I was not prepared, but I decided that I could accept the feelings and reject them as being true. I asked myself, if I let this thought be true, would it help me reach my goals? Because the answer was no, I rejected the truth of it.

I encourage this four-step process:

1. Identify the thought.

2. Accept that you have the thought.

3. Ask yourself, if I let this thought guide my behavior, will it help me be the best version of myself.

4. If no, reject it as a guiding force.

Defusion

Defusion is more of a process than a technique. It works in tandem with experiential acceptance. Cognitive fusion describes an attachment to negative thoughts as truth. When you experience fusion you see thoughts as absolute truths, as rules to follow, as threats, something you cannot let go of. Defusion means learning to step back from your thoughts. You recognize thoughts as something that may or may not be true or important and as non-threatening. Defusion reduces the negative impacts of thoughts on behavior. Take a step back and simply observe your thoughts instead of getting tangled up in them. Defusion will help you act more in line with your values, it will help you be more flexible in your decision making and will help you be less judgmental and more compassionate towards yourself.

Here is a drill you can use to separate yourself from your thoughts. You'll notice that by doing this you will achieve a sense of psychological distance from thoughts that weigh you down.

First, write down some of the negative thoughts that fill your mind: "I'm fat," "I'm lazy," "I'm out of shape."

Now reframe that thought by putting the phrase "I'm having the thought that…"

"I'm having the thought that I'm fat"

"I'm having the thought that I'm lazy"

"I'm having the thought that I'm out of shape"

Now let's take it one step further. Add "I notice" in front of the phrase.

"I notice I'm having the thought that I'm fat"

"I notice I'm having the thought that I'm lazy"

"I notice I'm having the thought that I'm out of shape"

Voila, you have achieved distance from the thoughts that make you feel less than capable to achieve your goals.

Urge Surfing

Urges are a natural response to strong habits or addictions. They are normal. Giving into urges can have negative impacts on goal attainment. Urge surfing is a technique that encourages you to treat urges like waves in the ocean.

The problem is when people give into urges before the intensity of the urge reduces. Urges increase in strength when you give into them. The more you accept and act on urges, the stronger and more frequent they will get, but when you successfully resist an urge, the opposite happens. Urges become less frequent and less intense. With urge surfing, you are encouraged to experience the urge as something that is brief, nonlethal, of relatively predictable course, and conquerable."

Think about the situations the lead up to having the urge. If the triggers are a situation, try not to put yourself in the urge producing situation. Make strategies to avoid or to cope with the triggers. Urge surfing, like psychological acceptance deals with being okay with discomfort.

IMPROVE CONFIDENCE AND CAPABILITIES AT THE RELATIONSHIP LEVEL

Hire a Coach

There is no point in suffering through second guessing what you are doing in the gym, or wondering if you are exercising properly, if the program you are on makes sense, or if you are eating the right foods. Not asking for help in the exercise realm is something that baffles me. If we have a health issue, we see a doctor, if it is time to do our taxes, we hire an accountant (thanks Dad), if we want to do renovations on our home, we hire a contractor. Trying to do any of these things on our own could prove to be a headache at best and disastrous at worse. We don't need this rugged individualism approach when it comes to our health. This is especially true with exercise or weight loss.

At some point it can become more expensive (and potentially dangerous) and frustrating to not hire a coach. I recently had a consult with a new client who was ready to get back into shape. He had been a member of Orange Theory and had tried online apps before. This is not a knock on any of these things, but large group classes and online apps don't provide you with feedback. This client had technique errors that if loaded or done under fatigue would cause unnecessary stress on his joints. Unfortunately (and not his fault), he had been doing exercises incorrectly for years.

With technical exercises like strength training (which is great for managing diabetes), you cannot add load on top of bad technique. The longer you exercise with poor technique the harder it is to unlearn. If you are unsure of yourself ask around for information on a reputable coach.

See Similar Others Succeed

When it comes to moderately risky things, I am a chicken. Recently I was in Vermont with my friend Patrick. We found a rope swing attached to a tree. Patrick is less risk averse than me. He climbed the tree and sat on a branch, grabbed the rope, and swung out into the lake. He landed in deep enough water, no problems. There is no way I would have been confident doing that until I saw someone else do it.

One of the sources of confidence is vicarious experience. Vicarious experience refers to the observation of people. Seeing people who are similar to ourselves succeed can increase our confidence that we also have the ability to succeed. We can feel more confident in starting new behaviors or reducing the frequency of problematic behaviors through observation and imitation of others.

Let's say you smoke, and you have three close friends who also smoke. You want to quit, and your friends also want to quit. Three of them begin the process of quitting and are successful. If you observe your three friends have success your confidence will also increase. The same concept goes for initiating health behaviors. Think of a friend who has turned their health around. What did they do? Ask them what worked for them to see if their methods are appealing.

Improve Confidence and Capabilities

Our environment promotes caloric intake and sedentary behavior. Obesity promoting, or obesogenic environments, like the one we live in, may be a driving force behind weight gain or inability to lose weight. People occupy numerous environments that be categorized as supportive or unsupportive[28] of health goals. Right now, we concern ourselves with environmental impacts on confidence and capabilities to engage in health behaviors.

When it comes to structural impacts on capabilities, we need to ask two questions: 1) does your current environment enable or disable the things that you want to do and 2) can we change it? If your environment thwarts your capabilities and you can change it, it is time to do just that. If it does not, then great, and if it does but you cannot change it, we need to explore alternative options. The goal of modifying your structural environment is to make the choice you want to make as close to unavoidable as possible.

Understanding the Built Environment

The built environment describes the physical design of the environment. Environments can be broken down into schools, workplaces, homes, and neighborhoods. Each comes with some level of control and modifiability. The built environment[28] has three factors: 1) physical design, 2) land use patterns, and 3) transportation systems.

Let's break it down. Imagine that you work 20 miles away from where you live. Your ability to actively commute to work is hindered. Now let's say you live one mile away from work in a nice neighborhood with sidewalks. You are much more likely to walk two miles each day. This is more of a recognition point. If your neighborhood does not have systems in place to promote physical activity you will need to find ways to do it yourself.

Defuse Disablers

Think of these structural factors as anything that is outside of your mind or your social network. Recently, I was out to dinner with some friends that were in town. The menu at the restaurant had the calories listed for their food. I was astonished that some meals were over 1,500 calories! This little piece of knowledge on the menu prompted me to act more knowledgably. My lack of knowledge about caloric content would have been a disabler to me making the best decision.

Let's continue with the example of eating because eating can be done for any number of reasons (hunger, hedonic pleasure, boredom, to relieve stress or anxiety, etc.). What environmental factors draw us away from eating how would like to eat? What disables or impairs our ability to self-regulate?

In a motor behavior class in my master's studies, I learned that it is impossible to pay full attention to two things at once. As in, there really is no such thing as good multitasking. A single task, such as eating, requires your full attention in order to be truly intentional. Eating of course is a social activity and we will never pay 100% attention to eating.

Reading, doing work, or watching television require attention as well. So, when you eat and watch television your attention is split. You are not processing all relevant information. In this sense, the television would be a structural disabler. It limits your capabilities to act intentionally and mindfully.

Dr. Marion Hetherington[29] from Glasgow Caledonian University conducted an eating experiment where participants ate food under different conditions. Participants ate alone, ate with other people, and ate while watching television. Food choice was evaluated using a buffet-style meal with different foods to choose from. Participants were able to choose from bread rolls filled with cheese, potato crisps, fresh green salad, coleslaw, and cakes. When participants ate in front of a television, they consumed 14% more calories than when they ate alone with no distractions. When eating, try to remove environmental distractors to eat more mindfully.

Make Enablers More Obvious

Before I moved to Boston, I spent my day in one building, often in one part of the building, the gym. When I worked as a strength coach at the State University of New York at Cortland I would just keep a gallon jug of water with me. By the end of the day, it should be gone (yes, I peed a lot), but when I moved to Boston, I had to do a lot of active commuting, bikes, walking, buses, trains. I was not too keen on carrying a gallon jug with me. The gallon jug worked out well because it was dichotomous, either I drank the gallon, or I did not. That feedback was motivating, and if I had some left at the end of the day, I would just drink it. In Boston I found myself drinking less water. That was until I moved and got a nice glass water container. Every night I cut up lemons or cucumbers and put them in the glass container to soak overnight. When I wake up, I have both tastier water and the return of feedback. Either the container is empty, or it is not. I ran into a barrier (active commuting) and came up with a solution to impact my behavior.

The environment should not thwart your abilities to do the things you want to do, it should promote them. An enabler would be a thing that would increase your confidence for a certain behavior. Along with opportunity, the available option must be something you are confident you can do. You can design a beautiful in-home gym but if you are not confident in your ability to use it, the opportunity factor does not matter.

Environmental adjustments to make the enablers more obvious (and the disablers less obvious) is going to be an ongoing process. To identify what enhances and what hampers your ability to be healthy, I want you to begin to self-monitor your behaviors. Self-monitoring is a behavior change strategy that is used to help self-regulate behavior. It is used to ensure that we do the things we intend to do (i.e. I intended to exercise three times this week, did I do it?). Self-monitoring is a motivational strategy, but it will help you identify triggers in your environment.

The structural environment is easier to change than the social environment. Here is what I recommend. First, identify what triggers unhealthy behaviors. You should use a chart like the one on the next page.

What did I do?	Where was I?	Who was I with?	What was I feeling?	Rank (-) ( ) (+)

Consider all the behaviors you engage in daily. By examining where you were and who you were with can help give insight as to what is influencing your behavior. Is it social or structural? What was the trigger. If it was the environment, change it. If the snacks in the fridge were the trigger, consider making them less accessible and visible or get rid of them. If it was social, consider the previous section on coping planning. Decide how you will act ahead of time in social situations.

USING THE 12-WEEK BEHAVIOR CHANGE WORKSHEET

This is what I am going to leave you with. In the next 12 weeks you are going to make whatever changes you want. Revisit the chart at the end of this chapter. First, clarify what you want out of your life and how your health and fitness relate to that. What is your health and fitness aspiration? Describe the best version of you. What are you doing? What do you look like? How do you feel? Then write down what you want to be doing consistently three months from now. What will the outcome be three months from now?

Then, think about what you would like to be doing this week. Pick behaviors that relate to your 12-week goal. What are you confident about and willing to do this week? When you write down your weekly goals ask yourself, what needs to be in place for me to be successful with this behavior? After the week is up revisit your behavioral goals. For each goal, what percent of success do you feel like you experience? Then what did you learn from your experience and how will you apply it to the next week? Then repeat the process. If you want to stick with your behavioral goals, great! If you need to make them easier or if you want to make it more challenging, then go ahead and do that. Pick what you think will be most successful and use the lessons you learned in this book to set yourself up for success. Specifically, if an issue comes up, examine, and fix your system. Was it a motivation, opportunity, or capability issue, and what caused the issue? What needs to change to make sure the issue does not happen again the next week? I promise if you follow this as is you will find success.

AFTERWORD

IN A RECENT CONVERSATION, A NEW CLIENT TOLD ME that he wanted to start making new healthy habits. He wanted them to stick because now was the time. He wasn't sick or limited, he just recognized if he continued down the path, he was going, it would not lead to the life he wanted.

So many of us either have health problems or are going down the route of having future health problems. Despite all the knowledge at our fingertips, our unhealthy lifestyles place us at serious risk. We continue with our unhealthy habits or seek out quick fixes only to be discouraged when they do not work. We come up short and we lose the confidence to continue. You might feel stuck, trying to navigate the obstacles and confusion related to health and wellness.

I believe that most people want to have health and fitness. They want to feel in control, to feel better, to have more balance, and confidence. However, I also recognize that there is a gap between what we want and what we have. I believe this book has laid out the groundwork for you to take control of your health. I believe that if you use the knowledge laid out in this book that you can find what works for you.

ABOUT THE AUTHOR

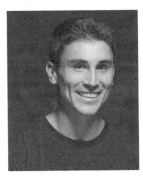

Justin Kompf, PhD, has worked in the fitness industry since 2009 as a college strength and conditioning coach and personal trainer. He has an MS in Exercise Science and has a PhD in Exercise and Health Sciences with a focus on Health Behavior Change from the University of Massachusetts at Boston. Justin has taught at the State University of New York at Cortland and also at the University of Massachusetts at Boston. He has published work in the *Strength and Conditioning Journal, Sports Medicine,* the *Journal of Physical Activity and Health*, and the *American Journal of Lifestyle Medicine.* He has contributed his expertise in health behavior change to personal training certifications and nutrition certifications with the National Academy of Sports Medicine.

REFERENCES

PREFACE

1. "What Is Diabetes?" Centers for Disease Control and Prevention. Centers for Disease Control and Prevention, June 11, 2020. https://www.cdc.gov/diabetes/basics/diabetes.html.

2. Colberg, Sheri et al. Exercise and type 2 diabetes: The American College of Sports Medicine and the American Diabetes Association: Joint position statement. *Diabetes Care* 33 (2010), 12: 147-167.

3. Forouhi, Nita., Misra, Anoop., Mohan, Viswanathan., Taylor, Roy. Dietary and nutritional approaches for prevention and management of type 2 diabetes. *The BMJ* 361 (2018), doi: 10.1136/bmj.k2234.

4. Papamichou, D., Panagiotakos, D., Itsiopoulos, I. Dietary patterns and management of type 2 diabetes: A systematic review of randomized clinical trials. *Nutrition, Metabolism, and Cardiovascular Diseases*. 29 (2019), 6: 531-543.

INTRODUCTION

1. Best Diets Overall. (2020). from https://health.usnews.com/best-diet/best-diets-overall

2. de Ridder, D., Adriaanse, M., Evers, C., Verhoeven, A. Who diets? Most people and especially when they worry about food. Appetite.80 (2014), 103-108.

3. Hales., C.M. et al. Prevalence of obesity among adults: United States, 2017-2018. NCHS Data Brief. 360. (2020).

4. Laycock, R., Choi, C. Americans spending 1.8 billion on unused gym memberships annually (2019). https://www.finder.com/unused-gym-memberships

5. Jean-Denis, G., Aliz, M., Pierre-Carl, M. Health club attendance, expectations, and self-control. Center for Economic Studies and ifo Institute. 4926. (2014).

6. Kearney, M.H., O'Sullivan J. (2003). Identity shifts as turning points in health behavior change. Western Journal of Nursing Research. 25 (2003) 2: 134-152.

7. 80 Year Old Powerlifting Grandma Shirley Webb Can Deadlift 255 Pounds. https://www.youtube.com/watch?v=cX4VNXnD0Dc

8. Michie, S., van Stalen, M.M., West, R. The behaviour change wheel: A new method for characterizing and designing behaviour change interventions. Implementation Science. 6 (2011): 42. doi: 10.1186/1748-5908-6-42

9. Heath, D. (2020). *Upstream*. Simon & Schuster.

CHAPTER 1

1. Faries., M.D. (2016). Why we don't "Just Do It": Understanding the intention-behavior gap in lifestyle medicine. American Journal of Lifestyle Medicine. 10 (2016), 322-329.

2. Rhodes, R.E., de Bruijn, G. How big is the physical activity intention-behaviour gap? A meta-analysis using the action control framework. British Journal of Health Psychology. 18(2013), 2, 296-309.

3. Jean-Denis, G., Aliz, M., Pierre-Carl, M. Health club attendance, expectations, and self-control. Center for Economic Studies and ifo Institute. 4926. (2014).

4. Godin-Gaston., Conner, M. (2008). Intention-behavior relationship based on epidemiologic indices: An application to physical activity. American Journal of Health Promotion. 22 (2008) 3: 180-182.

5. Ingledew, D.K., Markland, D. The role of motives in exercise participation. Psychology & Health. 23 (2008) 807-828.

6. Hunt, C. How Chris Pratt dropped 60 pounds in 6 months for 'guardians of the Galaxy'. Retrieved March 04, 2021, from https://www.mensjournal.com/health-fitness/how-chris-pratt-dropped-60-pounds-six-months/

7. Parks, L., Guay, R.P. Personality, values, and motivation. Personality and Individual Differences. 47 (2009), 675-684.

8. Forman, E.M., Butryn, M.L. A new look at the science of weight control: How acceptance and commitment strategies can address the challenge of self-regulation. Appetite. 84 (2015): 171-180.

9. Harris, R. ACT made simple: An easy-to-read primer on acceptance and commitment therapy. Oakland, CA: New Harbinger (2009).

10. Anderson, E. et al. Self-regulation, self-efficacy, outcome expectations, and social support: Social cognitive theory and nutrition behavior. The Society of Behavioral Medicine. (2007), 304-312.

11. Williams, D.M., Anderson, E.S., Winett, R.A. (2005). A review of the outcome expectancy construct in physical activity research. Annals of Behavioral Medicine. 29 (2005),1: 70-79.

12. Webb, T. The road to Hell, from https://www.psychologytoday.com/us/blog/the-road-hell/201608/the-road-hell.

13. de Ridder, D.T., de Wit, J.B. (2006). Self-regulation in Health Behavior. John Wiley & Sons Ltd.

14. Oettingen, G. (2015). *Rethinking positive thinking: Inside the new science of motivation.* New York, NY.

15. Rutledge, T. Why psychology trumps diet and exercise for weight loss. (2019). https://www.psychologytoday.com/us/blog/the-healthy-journey/201907/why-psychology-trumps-diet-and-exercise-weight-loss

CHAPTER 2

1. Goldberg, E. "This 99-year-old man begs every day and gives it all away to churches and orphanages. (2014) https://www.huffpost.com/entry/dobri-dobrev_n_4867974

2. Seligman, M. Learned helplessness. Annual Review of Medicine. 7050 (1972): 407-414.

3. Peterson, C. The future of optimism. American Psychologist. 55 (2000) 44-55.

4. Selva, Joaquin. Albert Ellis' ABC Model in the Cognitive Behavioral Therapy Spotlight. https://positivepsychology.com/albert-ellis-abc-model-rebt-cbt/

5. Peters, M.L., Flink, I., Boersma, K., Linton, S.J. Manipulating optimism: Can imagining a best possible self be used to increase positive future expectancies? The Journal of Positive Psychology. 5 (2010) 3: 204-211.

6. Michie, S., van Stalen, M.M., West, R. (2011). The behaviour change wheel: A new method for characterising and designing behaviour change interventions. Implementation Science. 42 (2011).

7. Rhodes, R.E., Williams, D.M., Mistry, C.D. Using short vignettes to disentangle perceived capability from motivation: A test using walking and resistance training behaviors. Psychology, Health & Medicine. 21 (2016) (5), 639-651.

CHAPTER 3

1. Scipioni, J.. Inside ex-bodybuilder Arnold Schwarzenegger's wellness routine now that he's 72.(2019). https://www.cnbc.com/2019/09/20/ex-bodybuilder-arnold-schwarzeneggers-wellness-routine-at-age-72.html

2. Verplanken. B. Sui, J. (2019). Habit and Identity: Behavioral cognitive, affective, and motivational facets of an integrated self. Frontiers in Psychology. 2019, 10, 1504.

CHAPTER 4

1. Locke, E.A., Latham G.P. (2002). Building a practically useful theory of goal setting and task motivation: A 35-year odyssey. American Psychologist 57(9), 705-717.

2. BJ Foggs book 'Tiny Habits'

3. Center for School Transformation

CHAPTER 5

1. Ryan, R.M., Deci, E.L. Self-Determination Theory: Basic Psychological Needs in Motivation, Development and Wellness. New York: The Guilford Press, 2018.

CHAPTER 6

1. Michie, S. van Stralen, M.M., West, R. The behaviour change wheel: A new method for characterizing and designing behaviour change interventions. Implementation Science. 2011, 6:42.

2.   Wood, W. Good Habits, Bad Habits: The Science of Making Positive Changes that Stick. London: Macmillan, 2019.

3.   Sallis, J.F. et al. The role of built environments in physical activity, obesity, and CVD. Circulation. 2013, 125(5): 729-737.

4.   Heath, C., Heath D. Switch: How to Change Things When Change is Hard. Random House, 2013.

5.   Friese, M., Hofmann, W., Wiers, R.W. On taming horses and strengthening riders: Recent developments in research on interventions to improve self-control in health behaviors. 2011, 336-351.

6.   Ritchie, C.. Fresh starts, guilty pleasures, and other pro tips for sticking to good habits. (2019). https://www.npr.org/sections/health-shots/2019/08/16/747332849/fresh-starts-guilty-pleasures-and-other-pro-tips-for-sticking-to-good-habits

7.   Bouton, M.E. Why behavior change is difficult to sustain. Preventative Medicine. 2014, 29-36.

8.   Godoy, M. 'Tiny Habits' are the key to behavioral change. 2020. https://www.npr.org/2020/02/25/809256398/tiny-habits-are-the-key-to-behavioral-change

9.   Welch, S. The rule of 10-10-10. 2006. https://www.oprah.com/spirit/suzy-welchs-rule-of-10-10-10-decision-making-guide/all

10. Miller, W.R., Rollnick, S. Motivational Interviewing: Preparing People for Change. New York. Guilford Press, 2002.

11. Clear, J. "How to stop procrastinating on your goals by using the "Seinfeld Strategy." https://jamesclear.com/stop-procrastinating-seinfeld-strategy.

12. Weinschenk, S. The power of the word 'because' to get people to do stuff (2013). https://www.psychologytoday.com/us/blog/brain-wise/201310/the-power-the-word-because-get-people-do-stuff

13. Rackow, P., Scholz, U., Hornung, R. Received social support and exercising: An intervention study to test the enabling hypothesis. British Journal of Health Psychology (2015) 20, 763-776.

14. Christakis, N.A., Fowler, J.H. The spread of obesity in a large social network over 32 years. The New England Journal of Medicine. 2007, 357: 370-379.

15. Cialdini, R.B., Kallgren, C.A., Reno, R.R. A focus theory of normative conduct: A theoretical refinement and reevaluation of the role of norms in human behavior. In M. P. Zanna (Ed.), Advances in experimental social psychology (Vol. 24, pp. 201–234). New York: Academic PressAdvances in Experimental Social Psychology. 1991,

16. de Castro, J.M., Brewer, E.M. The amount eaten in meals by humans is a power function of the number of people present. Physiology & Behavior. 1992, 51(1): 121-125.

17. Sallis, J.F., Glanz, K. Physical activity and food environments: Solutions to the obesity epidemic. 2009, 87(1), 123-154.

18. Vaccaro, A. She wants you to feel better about biking and walking in Boston. 2020. https://www.bostonglobe.com/business/2020/01/21/she-wants-you-feel-better-about-biking-and-walking-boston/Mtq9sVLR1L71rMjylbTZgL/story.html

19. Bauman et al., (2012). Correlates of physical activity: Why are some people physically active and others not? The Lancet. 380(9838). 258-271.

20. Kroese, F.M., Marchiori, D.R., de Ridder, D.T. Nudging healthy food choices: A field experiment at the train station. Journal of Public Health. 2016, 38(2): 133-137.

21. Laskey, J. (2020). What is 'self-nudging'? A simple trick to make healthier choices. 2020. https://www.today.com/health/what-self-nudging-simple-trick-make-healthier-choices-t184571

22. Cadario, R., Chandon, P. (2019). Which healthy eating nudges work best? A meta-analysis of field experiments. Marketing Science, 1-54.

23. Wansink, B., Painter, J.E., North, J. Bottomless bowls: Why visual cues of portion size may influence intake. Obesity research. 2005, 13(1): 93-100.

24. Sniehotta, F.F., Schwarzer, R., Scholz, U., Schuz, B. Action planning and coping planning for long-term lifestyle change: Theory and assessment. European Journal of Social Psychology. 2005, European Journal of Social Psychology, 35, 565-576.

25. Raynor, D.A., Coleman, K.J., Epstein, L.H. Effects of proximity on the choice to be physically active or sedentary. Research Quarterly in Exercise and Sport. 1998, 69(1): 99-103.

26. Bandura, A et al. Relative efficacy of desensitization and modeling approaches for inducing behavioral, affective, and attitudinal changes. Journal of Personality and Social Psychology. 1969, 13(3): 173-199.

27. Ross, L. The intuitive psychologist and his shortcomings: Distortions in the attribution process. In L. Berkowitz (Ed.), Advances in experimental social psychology. New York: Academic Press, in press

28. Lake, A., Townshend, T. Obesogenic environments: Exploring the built and food environments. 2006, 126 (6), 62-267.

29. Hetherington, M.M., Anderson, A.S., Norton, G.N., Newson, L. Situational effects on meal intake: A comparison of eating alone and eating with others. Physiology & Behavior. 2006, 30(4-5): 498-505.

NOTES

NOTES

NOTES

NOTES

NOTES

NOTES